The Headache & Neck Pain Workbook

AN INTEGRATED MIND AND BODY PROGRAM

Douglas E. DeGood, Ph.D.

Donald C. Manning, M.D., Ph.D.
and Susan J. Middaugh, Ph.D.

WITH A FOREWORD BY
Terence C. Davies, M.D.

NEW HARBINGER PUBLICATIONS

We would like to thank Panasonic Home and Commercial Products for permission to use the photo of the Panasonic Reach Easy Muscle Massager; the RoLoke Company for permission to use the illustration of the 4-in-1 WAL-PIL-O; and BodyCare, Inc. for permission to use the Posture Curve Lumbar Cushion illustration. Figures 6.3, 6.8, 6.9, 6.10, 6.11, and 6.16 are reprinted with permission from Visual Health Information (800-352-0709).

Publisher's Note

This publication is designed to provide accurate and authoritative information in regard to the subject matter covered. It is sold with the understanding that the publisher is not engaged in rendering psychological, financial, legal, or other professional services. If expert assistance or counseling is needed, the services of a competent professional should be sought.

Distributed in the U.S.A. by Publishers Group West; in Canada by Raincoast Books; in Great Britain by Airlift Book Company, Ltd.; in South Africa by Real Books, Ltd.; in Australia by Boobook; and in New Zealand by Tandem Press.

Cover design by Poulson/Gluck Design.
Text design by Tracy Marie Powell.
Edited by Catharine Sutker.

Illustrations 2.3, 5.1, 6.5, 6.7, 6.12, 6.13, 6.14, 6.15, 6.17a, and 6.17b by Seventeenth Street Studios. Illustrations 4.2, 4.4, 7.1, and A.1 by Valerie Winemiller.

Library of Congress Catalog Card Number: 97-66083

ISBN 1-57224-086-5

New Harbinger Publications' Web site address: www.newharbinger.com.

First Printing

This book is dedicated to my wonderful wife Drene.
Although challenged by headaches herself,
she has never been a "headache" to me.

—D. DeGood

Contents

Foreword

On the surface, this is a book about headaches; in reality, it is about many other things as well. The underlying theme is the practice of behavioral medicine, which is a sophisticated, scientific field with an impressive degree of proven success. Regrettably, for a variety of unfortunate reasons, the achievements of behavioral medicine have escaped the attention of most physicians. The information contained in these pages is therefore of compelling importance to doctors and patients alike.

In constructing this text, Dr. DeGood has demonstrated a special talent. The major challenge for any scientific author is to communicate his or her message effectively to a chosen audience. If the interpretation is too simplistic it will insult; if it is too scholarly, it will bore. This book bridges that gap. It will be read with pleasure and profit by both patients and practitioners. Predictably, when its principles are applied, it will enhance the well-being and quality of life of everyone who has the discipline to follow its precepts. It is my great hope that this text will be recognized by primary care practitioners for what it is, namely, a powerful aid with great potential for helping some of their distressed and difficult-to-treat patients.

Twentieth-century scientific medicine has established an amazing record of accomplishments. Its achievements have been so remarkable that patients can hardly be blamed for believing that there is a cure for every ailment. Of course, this belief is not true; in reality, medical treatments today have been estimated as offering cure (in the true sense of that word) to not more than 20 percent of all the illnesses that doctors treat. The vast bulk of illness is of the chronic variety and, by definition, is an incurable state of affairs. The medical task here is not to cure but to find ways to prevent, restrict, and ameliorate the progress of disease. The scientific method was not designed for this purpose, and so the management of most chronic illnesses remains in a state of incomplete resolution.

Frustrated by these shortcomings, innumerable patients with chronic illnesses (such as some varieties of headache) have sought relief outside the boundaries of conventional medicine. As a consequence, in recent years more patients have visited the offices of "alternative health care providers" than have consulted allopathic physicians. Alternative therapies, such as acupuncture and spinal manipulation, have attracted enthusiastic attention, with claims of benefit ranging from dramatic relief of infirmities to miraculous cures. Unhappily, the kind of rigorous proof that is demanded by the conventional medical establishment is usually lacking for these "alternative" outcomes. Behavioral medicine is the notable exception, inasmuch as it has scientific evidence of its effectiveness that goes back for at least a century.

Indeed, far from being "alternative," behavioral medicine needs to be recognized as an essential component of any *comprehensive* diagnostic and therapeutic plan that seeks to deal with chronic illness. Practitioners from some branches of contemporary medicine, including the field of family medicine, have advocated using behavioral medicine in any kind of clinical practice. In this context, it is noteworthy that Dr. DeGood himself works within one of the most conventional and prestigious medical institutions in this country. Clearly, the value of behavioral medicine is being recognized by some of the medical establishment's leadership.

As Dr. DeGood so carefully describes, the principles and practices of self-regulation are the keys to effective behavioral medicine. Self-regulation requires that patients learn to regain control of their state of well-being. The clinician's task is to facilitate the patients' progress toward acquiring dominance over their physical symptoms. Philosophically, we can reflect that this is the overriding desire of every patient, namely to retain or regain "control." Despair over the loss of control and the consequent sense of vulnerability, have been recognized as the primary stigmata of patienthood. Once sensed as impending, most people will strive to avoid such a state of affairs. Self-regulation is not easy; it requires the kind of commitment that only very determined patients are willing to bring to bear to gain control over their symptoms.

Some thirty years ago, Dr. Kerr White described features of "The Ecology of Illness" in a paper that was published in the *New England Journal of Medicine*. It was Dr. White's observation that in any given month, twice as many people become ill as the number who seek assistance from physicians. In other words, most people manage to take care of themselves and avoid going to doctors. Self-care takes many forms, and patient diaries reveal everything from going shopping for new clothes as a distraction from symptoms, to seeking the advice of a friend or neighbor. Some of this activity may involve denial of disease or fear of what a visit to a physician may reveal. There can be little doubt, however, that people are actively seeking ways to become more self-efficacious. The boom in self-help texts and audiovisual products that has been evolving for the past couple of decades is dramatic evidence of this trend.

The movement towards self-help has been heightened by an increasing realization of the benefits of preventing illness. Once the concept of health risk has been recognized, it is virtually impossible for any intelligent person to ignore the fact that at least 50 percent of all disease and untimely death is linked to unhealthy lifestyles. Additionally, and perhaps most significantly, people have become increasingly aware of the significance of the mind-body interface. The fact that the mind and body are not only inseparable but exquisitely interactive has been avoided if not denied ever since Descartes proclaimed the mind-body dichotomy. At last, there is evidence of a dawning, popular realization that personal destiny ultimately may be influenced by willful thinking; and this, of course, is the keystone principle of applied psychophysiology, which is the scientific basis of self-regulation.

There are good reasons to believe that the time is ripe for this text. If it is appreciated and its principles are widely applied, then I predict with a high degree of certainty that we can anticipate a seachange in the conventional approaches to managing chronic illness.

—Terence C. Davies, M.D.
Professor and Chairperson,
Department of Family and Community Medicine
Eastern Virginia Medical School,
Glenn R. Mitchell Chair of Generalist Medicine

Preface

Although this book is primarily about headaches, the word "neck" is included in the title because structures in the neck often contribute to the headache syndrome. This book is not about neck problems that stem from injury or degenerative disease of the cervical spine and adjacent tissues, which may cause neck pain independent of headaches. To avoid the tedium of constantly repeating the term "headache and neck pain," the generic term "headache" will be used, and it should be understood to include neck pain.

The chief goal of this workbook is to teach you how to use psychophysiologic self-regulating skills as a part of a comprehensive plan for managing your headaches. In addition to self-regulation, the other two components of this comprehensive plan are medication and exercise/physical therapy. These latter two are covered by Donald C. Manning, M.D., in chapter 8, and Susan J. Middaugh, Ph.D., in chapter 6.

The theme that dominates this workbook is how to learn self-regulating techniques—using your own cognitions (attention and thoughts) to monitor and regulate physiologic change in your body in the direction of pain reduction and physiological calming. Few of these techniques are unique to headache management; rather they are general stress and pain management strategies as applied to headaches.

I hope you will find that this book takes some of the mystery out of psychophysiologic self-regulation. Efforts have been made to reduce self-regulating exercises to a few basic components, and to represent these by easy-to-remember key words. These key words are memory cues to guide your self-regulating efforts.

No matter how serious your headaches are, I believe you will find that the self-regulation techniques will make a difference in the way you respond to them, and hopefully, in time, will reduce their frequency and severity. The sooner you get started learning self-regulating skills the better. If your headaches are only a minor problem, with these techniques you may be able to avoid a future of escalating problems. Even if you continue to need medications for your headaches, knowing how to use self-regulation techniques can make headache management easier both for you and your doctor.

Chapters 1, 2, and 3 contain considerable information and theory about the physiological underpinnings of headaches and self-regulation techniques. Theoretically you could skip these chapters and move directly to working with the basic self-regulating skills described in chapters 4, 5, and 6. But I urge you to read this background information because the better you understand the physiology of stress and headaches, the more logical and interesting you will find your efforts at self-regulation.

Once you become familiar with the psychophysiologic self-regulation techniques described in chapters 4 and 5, you'll be able to use the remaining chapters to supplement and polish your basic skills. Certainly the strategic use of medications (chapter 8) and the development of correct posture and muscle functioning (chapter 6) can greatly aid you in controlling your headaches. Chapter 7 will acquaint you with biofeedback, an interesting, relatively new technology for teaching self-regulation. Chapter 9 addresses the fact that for some people controlling their headaches will require not only alterations in their physical response to stressors, but may also require addressing the *causes* of those stressors. The final chapter puts all these ideas together in what I hope will become for you a straightforward, effective plan for coping with your headaches.

The primary focus of this book is self-regulation of headaches. There are also more comprehensive resource books available for information on the possible causes, diagnosis, and medical management of headaches. Some of these books are listed under "Further Reading" in the various chapters.

Finally, it is my hope to provide you with more than just facts about headaches. I also want to encourage you to develop patience and persistence in taking control of your headaches. Self-regulation is not just a set of exercises; it is also an attitude, a way of thinking about our relationship to pain and illness.

—Douglas E. DeGood, Ph.D.

I would like to thank my many colleagues and students at the University of Virginia Pain Management Center, as well as the patients, who have made all my efforts at teaching self-management training possible. Special thanks go to Lee Adams, LPC and Biofeedback Therapist, who has played a vital role in our headache and neck pain program, and to Joseph Dane, Ph.D., who has done much to enhance my knowledge and appreciation of the interaction between mind and body. Additionally, I would like to thank Kristin Beck, Acquisitions Editor, Kayla Sussell, Developmental Editor, and Catharine Sutker, Copy Editor, of New Harbinger Publications for their valuable support and assistance with this project.

CHAPTER 1

What Can You Do About Your Headaches?

▲ Benign headaches vs. serious underlying problem

▲ Stress-related headaches

▲ What is a self-regulation strategy?

▲ A comprehensive treatment plan

▲ There is hope!

Headache! The word itself suggests pain and stress, or insurmountable frustration—as in "this job, person, or situation is such a headache." That's the way most people with frequent headaches experience their discomfort; as an irritating frustration they just have to put up with along with all the other stresses of life.

Probably a headache is the one chronic pain condition that most of us associate with everyday physical and emotional tension. Many of you may already know that headaches are a most peculiar type of pain in that they are usually *benign*—that is, not symptomatic of serious injury, disease, or some other lasting tissue damage. That is, a headache is seldom life threatening. Most often tension, stress, and/or some other headache trigger affect the nerves, muscles, and blood vessels of the head and neck in such a way as to cause pain. Most of you have almost certainly noticed the discomfort that can affect your back, neck, and shoulder muscles with tension, fatigue, and overexertion. Sometimes a pattern of frequent headaches may start with a minor injury to the head or neck. Even though the injury itself may not have been serious and recovery seems to have taken place, the headache pattern may persist.

There are a few noteworthy exceptions to the benign status of headaches. Headaches can be secondary to serious traumatic head and neck injury, or to quite a number of serious illnesses. High blood pressure, fever, or any physical event that changes the pressure of the circulating cerebral spinal fluid can cause headaches. Finally, headaches are a common symptom of tissue damage resulting from tumors, strokes, or more rarely, intercranial infections. Anyone who develops headaches for the first time or experiences an abrupt change in their headache symptoms' pattern should be medically evaluated before beginning any treatment plan. Whenever a headache or neck pain is symptomatic of a serious underlying physical problem, the pain is fulfilling its proper role of alerting the individual to the presence of a problem that may threaten survival. This book is not about such pain, but rather about the vast majority (95 percent) of head and neck pain that falls into the benign category, i.e., where the pain alarm mechanisms work more like a "false alarm" producing pain sensations with no particular survival value.

The Frustrating Odyssey of the Headache Patient

Many readers already will be familiar with a frustrating sequence of events that can follow the onset of chronic benign headaches. You may have found yourself becoming gradually concerned by the increasing frequency and intensity of reoccurring headaches. Your efforts to control your headache with over-the-counter medications seemed not to work. You made an appointment with a primary care physician, and he or she conducted a physical exam and requested blood tests to rule out more general underlying causes, such as a viral infection or blood glucose irregularities. Finding nothing suspicious, your physician made a diagnosis of a common headache pattern such as tension, migraine, or mixed headache and prescribed a medication; for example, Fiorinal is currently one of the most popular. If your severe headache pain is only occasional, your doctor may not have hesitated to prescribe a painkiller, such as Percocet® or Vicodin®. However, if your headaches persisted, worsened, or the medication lost its effectiveness, you were probably referred to a headache specialist, usually a neurologist. The neurologist may have done a brain and upper spinal cord imaging—Xray, CT (computerized axial tomography), PET (position emission tomography), or MRI (magnetic resonance imaging)—looking for evidence of tumors, blood vessel bulges or leaks, or any other evidence of structural irregularity in the brain or spinal cord. When nothing suspicious was found, a new round of medications was tried. In time, if this form of management was unsuccessful, you may have been referred to other specialists.

A common pattern in severe cases is that new medications help for a while, but over time they seem to lose effectiveness, leaving the patient in worse pain than ever. This is because medications, while providing temporary relief, may actually interfere with long-term tolerance of pain. As a last resort, you may have been referred to a specialized comprehensive pain center or to a headache clinic. It is in this type of clinic that a headache patient may first be exposed to alternative therapies, especially the self-regulation therapies described in this book.

For many patients it is unfortunate that exposure to these therapies doesn't come earlier, preferably in the primary care setting. That's because the headache pattern is more readily amenable to self-regulation at an earlier stage.

You may feel a certain amount of frustration with doctors who dismiss headache complaints rather casually once serious underlying pathology has been ruled out. The message seems to be that because the condition is not life threatening, you shouldn't worry about it and should just ignore it. But it is far easier for the doctor to dismiss the pain than it is for the headache sufferer to do so. In fact, an intense migraine headache may be the worst pain you can possibly experience without it being a warning of a serious underlying physical problem. Or, a more sophisticated, well-meaning doctor may say that it's just a stress-related problem and suggest that you try to reduce the stress in your life. However, the connection to stress may be very ambiguous, and even if so, how are you suppose to reduce your level of stress?

Headaches and the Stress of Life

Patients sometimes feel uneasy when doctors say that their headaches might be "stress related." They may feel greater unease if "stress management" or other behavioral-based "relaxation" techniques are suggested as an alternative to medication. Many of you will recognize these as "psychological" techniques and therefore may feel that if such procedures can help you, your headache is not quite "legitimate." Since most headaches are not associated with lasting tissue damage, and can be helped by stress-management techniques, does that mean that they are "imaginary" psychological events without an actual physical basis?

Clearly, the answer is no. Even if a headache is a response to stress, very real physical events are involved. If you have repeated benign (not life threatening) headaches, it is likely that you have a biological tendency toward some biochemical or neurological disturbance of the brain or surrounding tissue structures. This tendency, in turn, is set into action by some physical, emotional, or environmental triggering mechanism, or a combination of such triggers. These triggers are called *stressors*, and our physical and emotional reactions are called *stress* or *stress reactions*. Stressors may be serious losses or threats to our well-being, but they also can include simply keeping up with a demanding daily schedule. Also, remember that stressors need not be experienced only as negatives. Positive events, e.g., a job promotion, a child's wedding, or taking a vacation, may still be stressful to your physical systems even when you are enjoying yourselves. Recall your having to "recover" from a fun-packed but strenuous vacation or holiday.

The physical effects of stress on our neuroendocrine and muscular systems can be considerable. These reactions are normal, expected, and part of the biological fight-or-flight survival response that is discussed in chapter 4. Life can never be stress-free, nor would we want it to be. Stress in controlled amounts is seldom harmful. In fact, stress in controlled doses strengthens us physically and emotionally. Our lives would be pretty dull if we never faced any responsibilities or new challenges, never exercised, or sat on the edge our seats at sporting events. But when stressors are prolonged, or stress reactions continue well beyond the removal of the actual stressor, then we begin to risk the development of stress-related physical symptoms. Stress reactions that continue beyond the removal of the stressor may be commonplace, where for unknown or possibly genetic reasons our bodies overreact to the stressor events. Long after the argument, the work project, or final exam is over, the physical reaction may linger. Headaches can result from stressful events that seem to go on and on.

It is important not to think of stressors as some kind of evil forces that magically transform themselves into headaches. There is a complex set of physical reactions that transforms a stressor into a headache, although sometimes this transformation is so complex that the link between the stressor and the symptom is obscured. This is particularly the case with rebound migraine headaches where a pattern of physiological events leading to a headache may be triggered by stressors, but the headache itself appears only after the stressor is over. Such headaches are sometimes referred to as "weekend," "vacation," or even "relaxation" headaches. Furthermore, headache-producing stressors may interact with other triggers, such as alcohol, fatigue, hormonal changes, heat, or various foods and aromas. These common triggers may not elicit a headache every time, but may be more potent in the presence of stressor conditions. Figure 1.1 shows a model of some of the ways that stressors are related to headaches.

The components of the model are as follows:

Life stressors: These are the everyday demands of life. Some stressors are positive, pleasurable, or exciting. Mostly, however, they are those people or events around us that challenge our ability to cope, e.g., a sick child, a demanding boss, an unpaid tax bill, and so forth.

Personal perception of stressors: This is how we uniquely perceive or appraise the stressors in our lives. What they mean to you depends on your current circumstances and past experiences. Your perceptions can modify the strength and

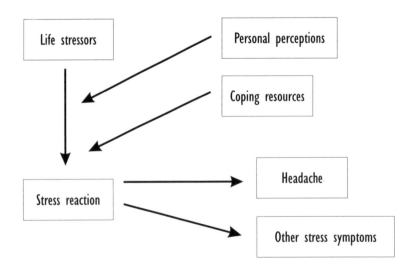

Figure 1.1:   **The Connection between Headaches and Stressors**

impact of a stressor. Also, certain personality traits, such as perfectionism, compulsiveness, and impatience, when carried to extremes, can add to stress.

Coping resources: These include the amount of control you have over the stressor; that is, can you change or modify it? They also include your ability to control (or self-regulate) your cognitive and physiological reactions to the stressor.

Stress or stress reactivity: These are your cognitive (thoughts and feelings) and physiological reactions to stressors. A headache can be just one aspect of your stress reactivity. Some people may have a genetic or acquired predisposition to respond to stressors with headaches; others may respond with stomach upset or back pain.

Figure 1.1 suggests that stressor events in our lives set off stress reactions, but that the severity of the reaction is not simply a result of the severity of the stressors. Your reaction to stressors can be modified by your personal perception of the stressors as well as by your coping resources. Coping resources in turn include both the capacity to control the stressors and the ability to control your cognitive and physiological reaction to the stress.

As you go through this workbook, you will notice that most of your attention will be directed to developing skills to control your reactions to stressors, with the exception of chapter 9, which addresses control of the stressors themselves. Even for headaches that may not be directly caused by stressors, headache pain itself can be a stressful event for which self-regulating skills can be helpful.

Comprehensive Headache Management Programs

The key goal of this book is to teach you how to use psychophysiologic self-regulation skills as part of a comprehensive headache management program.

A comprehensive headache management program must be one that you understand and with which you feel comfortable. It must provide you with a sense of control—a feeling that you know what to do to cope with your headaches. It usually will require a doctor who can regulate medication and help you coordinate the type of plan described in later chapters, involving medicine, physical therapy, and the use of self-regulating techniques.

This workbook will provide you with information about, and instructions for using, cognitive psychophysiologic self-regulation techniques for headaches. The term *cognitive* implies that the physiologic self-regulation you're trying to acquire is achieved by focusing your attention and thoughts. The term *psychophysiologic* means that your mind and body are working together in this effort. Other terms that you may already be familiar with, such as mental imagery, autogenic training, biofeedback, or progressive muscle relaxation, are all specific strategies to achieve psychophysiologic self-regulation. Sometimes these therapies are also classified as *behavioral therapies*, to distinguish them from other medical approaches. Note, however, that self-regulation strategies are just one of many forms of behavioral therapy.

It is part of our culture to believe that if you have a headache you should "take something for it." And if that doesn't work, you should see a doctor who can "give you something stronger." Certainly, medications have a role in a comprehensive management program, but there are other important strategies that can also help. With severe headaches, these alternatives will reduce the amount of medication you need to control them. In cases of mild headaches, the alternatives may actually eliminate them entirely.

What Is a Self-Regulation Strategy?

As the name implies, a self-regulation therapy is something you do yourself. The term also implies using the self (your attention, effort) to control physiological systems in your body, with the goal of achieving physical calming and reducing pain-impulse traffic in your nervous system.

We all recognize that our thoughts and feelings affect our bodies. Think of a time when you were frightened or anxious. Do you remember how you could feel your heart pounding and your jaw and chest muscles tightening? Were your hands cold and sweaty? Did your back ache? Fortunately, our thoughts and feelings also have the power to affect our bodies in the opposite direction, that is, to make us feel relaxed and comfortable. This positive capacity can be harnessed to help manage our headaches. This is what self-regulation is all about.

How can you learn to use self-regulation to control your headaches? It is important to understand that you must learn strategies to focus and quiet your mind so that you can relax and calm your body. Through using such self-control techniques as breath control, focused attention on muscle activity, and guided mental imagery, you can learn to increase your awareness of the subtle physiological changes that signal a more relaxed state. When mentally calm and physically relaxed, some people actually can learn to "turn down" their pain sensation, much as if they have taken an analgesic. Biofeedback is another way to assist with this process. These are all natural processes, well within the normal capacity of the mind and body, but few of us know, without training, how to use these inherent capacities fully.

Effectiveness of Self-Regulation for Headaches

The low risks involved—as well as the inherent appeal of self-regulating pain sensations without drugs or surgery—should make these techniques a desirable therapy. But many of you may be thinking: Can a treatment that depends on something I learn to do myself really be effective?

Multiple studies have indicated that 50 to 70 percent of headache patients benefit from these strategies, a figure very similar to the response to medication, but without the associated risk of side effects (Blanchard and Diamond 1996). An independent panel of the National Institutes of Health (1995) concluded that cognitive-behavioral self-regulation therapies are effective treatments for pain, especially headaches. Whether the benefits persist is not always clear, but with the efficacy of drug therapies notoriously short-lived, it's assumed that the benefits of learning self-regulating skills are at least as enduring as most drug treatments.

As is true of all headache treatments, the self-regulation techniques will be more effective for those with occasional mild or moderate headaches than for those with persistent severe headaches. Acquiring cognitive control over a psychophysiologic response habit is easier if done *before* the pattern is well-habituated. But all too often patients never hear about self-regulating alternatives for headaches until drug therapy has been exhausted or has led to drug tolerance or dependence. If self-regulation techniques were better understood and more widely available within primary care medical settings, such escalations might be prevented more frequently.

A Comprehensive Treatment Plan

How self-regulation learning will fit into an overall headache management plan will depend on the frequency and intensity of your headaches. Four different patterns of headaches are described below.

1. Occasional (Episodic) Mild Headache

    Most headaches are merely nuisances rather than life-disrupting. Such headaches diminish while you relax after a good meal or respond quickly to over-the-counter medication. Seeking a doctor for such headaches is unnecessary unless the headache pattern should change abruptly or suddenly be accompanied by strange neurological symptoms.

    Unfortunately, people who have severe headaches are more likely to read this workbook than those with mild ones. This is unfortunate because many of you with mild headaches probably could eliminate them completely by learning to voluntarily relax the muscles of your neck and head. Learning to control muscle tension habits while still relatively young, or when headaches are still mild, can provide lifelong benefits in the prevention of future headaches.

2. Occasional (Episodic) Severe Headache

    Some of you may experience very severe headaches but only occasionally—maybe three or four times a year, certainly not more than once a month. You should report this type of episodic headache to your doctor who often can make it more tolerable with medication. If you benefit from medication, or if the headaches never last for more than a day or two and seldom keep you from your normal activities, reliance on medication may be fine. But keeping in mind the potential of episodic severe headaches to increase in frequency over time, you might consider trying out some of the techniques described in this workbook. By adding self-regulating skills to your repertoire of options, you may be able to keep your headaches from escalating over time and to minimize your need for medication. When you do need medication, you can enhance its effects with self-regulation techniques. You can experiment with the ideas in this workbook on your own. Seek a referral to a teacher of self-regulation techniques only if you have difficulty learning these strategies.

3. Frequent Severe Headaches

    Some of you may experience severe headaches as often as two or three times a month. Headaches this frequent, if severe, can take a heavy toll on you at home or at work. You should definitely undergo a physical exam. A common sequence of events leading to this pattern is that of women who began with severe menstrual cycle–related headaches, but gradually the headaches began to escalate toward weekly intervals. Medication may give significant relief and provide adequate control for many years, but, eventually, the headaches may just become too frequent to be controlled by moderate amounts. Tolerance and/or dependency on medication may develop, and the medication must be switched frequently to maintain even moderate control over the headache. Eventually, medications may actually become part of the headache pattern itself—whenever the blood level of the medication drops significantly, the headache returns with full vigor. The concept of "rebound" headaches will be discussed in chapter 2. Obviously, this is a headache pattern that requires multidisciplinary effort beyond medication alone.

4. Continuous Headaches

Finally, a fourth headache pattern is that of the continuous or nearly continuous headache. This pattern comes in a variety of forms. Some people report that a low or moderate level headache is present all the time, with a more intense headache superimposed at various intervals. Others report an intense headache attack nearly every day, but not lasting all day. Still others report almost continuous, very severe headaches present nearly all the time, interrupted occasionally only for a day or two. No matter what the history, if headaches become this persistent, medical attention must be sought. If the diagnosis remains that of a benign headache condition, an initial period of withdrawal from all medications may be recommended to try to re-establish the true baseline headache activity. Usually some type of medication will then be reinstated, but it's hoped that the doctor will also recommend consultation with a behavioral headache management specialist familiar with the strategies described in this workbook. With this type headache pattern it would be very difficult for a patient to learn self-regulating techniques effectively without professional guidance.

Be Realistic—but Do Not Give Up!

Do not give up too easily on learning how to better control your headaches. Too often, a well-meaning advisor may say, "Try some relaxation tapes," without offering any further guidance. This may be a good starting point but it falls short of what is required. It is understandable that you may feel discouraged, or even skeptical, when all treatment efforts in the past, including past efforts at self-regulation, have led to failure. If you are one of those frustrated individuals, you may find it difficult to imagine that you can do anything yourself—especially by making some simple changes in your thoughts and behavior. But stay with it and look for small, gradual, incremental gains. If your headaches are severe and have been present for many years, it is likely to take weeks or even months before you begin to notice progress, and you will probably require some continuing use of medication. But remember that any positive improvement at all, even the slightest, is a step in the right direction. Like learning to ride a bicycle or play a musical instrument, these skills once acquired can continue to grow and be used indefinitely.

Key Word Summary

To ensure that you have thoroughly mastered the material in this chapter, write the definition of each term below in your own words. Future chapters will build on your understanding of these terms.

Stressor: _____

_____

_____

Personal perception: _____

_____

_____

Coping resources: _____

_____

_____

Stress reactivity: _____

_____

_____

Cognitive: _____

_____

_____

Psychophysiologic: _____

_____

_____

Self-regulation: _____

_____

_____

Further Reading

Blanchard, E. B. and F. Andrasik. 1985. *Management of Chronic Headache: A Psychological Approach*. Elmsford, NY: Pergamon Press.

Duckro, P. N., W. D. Richardson, and J. E. Marshall. 1995. *Taking Control of Your Headaches*. New York: Guilford Press.

Rapoport, A. M. and F. D. Sheftell. 1990. *Headache Relief*. New York: Simon & Schuster.

Chapter 2

How Headaches Work

▲ Structure of head and neck

▲ Predisposition toward headaches

▲ Headache triggers

▲ Physiology of headaches

▲ Types of headaches

This somewhat more technical chapter is included in this workbook because many readers find headaches to be terribly confusing and even mysterious. It seems almost impossible that pain can be this severe without anything being seriously wrong. This chapter will explain how this can be. An appreciation of the structure of the head and neck will help you grasp why head and neck pain can be so persistent as well as so difficult to diagnose and treat. Furthermore, if you understand some of the possible underlying causes of headaches, you will better understand the rationale behind many of the techniques and recommendations spelled out in this workbook.

Structure of the Head and Neck

After careful consideration of the structure of the head and neck, it seems remarkable that anyone ever manages to be headache-free. This particular region is one of the most complex and vulnerable parts of the body.

The neck is a narrow isthmus, crowded with crucial structures, connecting head to torso. All the information reaching the brain, and the returning neural signals that influence every part of the body, must pass through the cervical vertebrae (the neck bones of the spine) and into the base of the brain. Major arteries and veins pass through the neck, as do the trachea and esophagus. Squeezed in as well are the larynx (voice box), lymph nodes, and other glands. All of these critical structures are supported and held in place by multiple layers of muscles, tendons, and ligaments that attach to the base of the skull, to the spinal vertebrae, and to the other bones of the upper back and chest.

The head, which weighs about as much as a bowling ball, is perched on top of the spinal column, and those bony segments of the spine—the cervical vertebrae—are very small at the upper end. Imagine the tremendous pressure put on these vulnerable neck tissues when this "bowling ball" is uncontrollably projected by a fall or snapped by whiplash in a motor vehicle accident. It would be inevitable that such overstretching would lead to at least some tearing of muscles and nerves.

People who don't suffer from headaches tend not to think much about the structures covering the skull. Actually, there are very few pain-sensitive nerve endings inside the skull, but the thin layer of tissue surrounding the skull is richly supplied with nerve endings and blood vessels. What lies within this layer is the source of most of our headaches. For example, an important sensory nerve called the trigeminal nerve is found there. It is called "tri" because it has three main branches. It exits through small openings on either side of the skull and serves the head and upper chest area. Each branch has offshoots that run throughout the face and head and carry pain information from all over the head, the mucous membranes of the mouth, the teeth, and the sac surrounding the outer brain. With this kind of rich nerve supply, it is not surprising that the face and head are so sensitive to pain. This may also help you to understand how pain originating in one part of the head can be transferred easily to another part.

Muscle Irritation of the Neck and Head

Correct positioning and pain-free head movement depend on the complex layers of crisscrossing muscles and tendons of the neck. Compared to our awareness of neck muscles, we tend to be even less aware of the flat muscles over much of the face and head. But the face and scalp are not just skin over bone. Without these muscles and tendons, you could not chew, wrinkle your nose, purse your lips, raise your eyebrows, smile, or frown. If tense, these muscles, as well as the neck muscles, may become painful or indirectly cause pain by putting pressure on blood vessels and nerves.

To properly contract and extend, all these layers of muscles must slide and glide smoothly and comfortably. Otherwise, movement and posture of the head and upper body can't be maintained without discomfort. If you think about all the bending, contracting, and stretching involved in such a simple routine as rotating your head through a full 180-degrees, from side to side, it's remarkable that normally we have so little discomfort. Think of all those lubricated internal surfaces of bone, muscle, and tendon that must constantly rub over each other without irritation to accomplish basic motion. The potential for irritation is considerable, given even minor damage to a muscle or the tendons' connection to bones. That irritation can affect blood vessels and nerves, which can result in more irritation and pain. It's analogous to the discomfort a stray particle irritating your eyeball can cause. Many of these sources of pain are extremely difficult to pinpoint. Small patches of scar tissue may cause excessive friction between inner moving surfaces. Every bone and muscle in your body moves within a lubricated sheath. Anything that makes the tissues rub or stick together, or move without adequate lubrication, can cause irritation and pain.

All muscle action must be synchronized and balanced. If a muscle on one side of the head or neck is slightly weaker or less flexible than on the other side, it can create odd patterns of pain and produce wear and tear on adjacent joints and soft tissues, much as walking with a limp in one leg can produce pain in the other leg or the back.

Sometimes the aggravation can be pinpointed to sensitive or irritated spots in the muscle (called *trigger points*). Other times, muscle irritation can be a more generalized ache or discomfort without specific trigger points. See figure 2.1 for a picture of the complexity of the muscles in the head and neck.

Muscle Dysfunction and Headaches

When the muscles of the head and neck remain tight for prolonged periods of time, that tightness can lead to muscle tension headaches. Furthermore, the tight muscles can place pressure on the many nerves and blood vessels in this area. Today, many doctors and other headache specialists believe that nearly all headache types, including migraines, are triggered by muscle dysfunction. Although

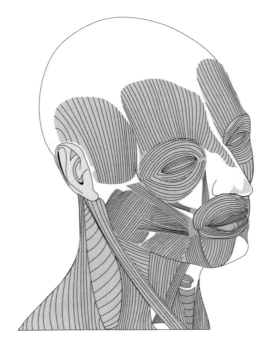

Figure 2.1:   **Muscles in the Head and Neck**

a migraine typically involves a complex set of neurochemical changes leading to painfully irritated blood vessels in the scalp, in some cases, the response may begin with irregular muscle functioning in the neck and head. Physical therapists have long known that some migraine patients respond well to physical manipulation of trigger points around the eyes, jaw muscles, and neck muscles.

Why are head and neck muscles so vulnerable to dysfunction? It's easy to understand pain that begins after a muscle injury caused by an accident. But many muscle problems may result simply from the wear and tear of normal living. How often do you bump your head, twist or overstretch your neck, squint your eyes, clench your jaw, grit your teeth, or chew gum or hard candy? That's a lot of wear and tear. Some therapists also suggest that poor posture plays an important part in head and neck pain. They point out that many people display an excessive forward head posture, where the weight of the head is not well balanced between the shoulders on the top of the spinal column, but instead extends forward. This creates a constant pulling pressure on the soft tissues at the back of the neck. This posture is commonplace in our society where so much of the work we do is at desks, tables, and benches, and requires a forward-leaning, head-down position. Eventually the head may become permanently locked in this posture and feel normal to the individual, but it places a chronic strain on the muscles, which eventually will rebel.

Predisposition Toward Headache and Headache Triggers

If you are hoping for a simple straightforward account of the causes of headaches you're going to be disappointed. The suspected causes are so numerous and complex that we can't talk about single causes but only about interacting events that result in headaches. The concept of interactions helps to explain the well-known unpredictability of headaches. No doubt some of you have had the experience that a certain food, aroma, or activity will sometimes, but not always, give you a headache. Likewise, removal of the headache trigger may not eliminate all headaches, and, gradually, headaches may return in response to a new trigger. It can be very frustrating when it seems that as soon the headaches are brought under control they reappear in some new form or with some new trigger. Such a pattern certainly suggests that for people with a strong predisposition for headaches, more than one cause can set off a headache.

Diathesis: A Predisposition to Headaches

In medicine, a constitutional predisposition to develop some symptom is called a *diathesis*. A diathesis is often genetic, but it can also be acquired by way of an accident, illness, or in another manner. Diatheses are very common, but do not always lead to symptoms. For example, although diabetes has a clear genetic link, not all children of diabetic parents develop the disorder. Expression of the diathesis for diabetes, i.e., actually becoming diabetic, may also depend on diet, weight, stress, smoking, or other general health factors.

Even though headaches, especially migraines, tend to run in families, it has been very difficult to determine the exact degree of genetic diathesis. The Canadian headache researcher David Bakal (1994) reports that some studies find that up to 80 percent of migraine sufferers have parents who have similar problems. He concludes, however, that better-designed studies of twins suggest that genetics actually may play only a very limited role in headache susceptibility. Bakal sites studies finding concordance rates (both twins have headaches) of around 27 percent for identical twins and 15 percent for nonidentical twins. If migraines were a pure product of genetic makeup, we would expect a 100 percent concordance rate among identical twins, with a much lower rate for nonidentical twins.

Bakal stresses that this twin data should help headache sufferers avoid feeling trapped by their genes, i.e., believing they have a predetermined condition about which they can do nothing. He further states that although there is no doubt that genetic factors contribute to the early development of headaches, once the disorder begins to increase in frequency, there are other important factors that determine whether it becomes a chronic problem. He proposes a psychophysiological model of headache development. The model states that one's physical and emotional reactions when headaches first begin to appear can set the stage for the pattern of future headaches. As they become more serious, both psychological and physiological reactions mutually reinforce each other in a downward spiral until finally the headaches seem to have an autonomy that appears to be independent of anything in the person's environment.

Headache Triggers

Reaction to a headache trigger is not usually an allergy but rather a sensitivity. For individuals who have a diathesis for headaches, some of the commonly reported headache triggers are the following:

- psychological stress
- alcohol
- certain foods
- irregular sleep
- for women, hormonal fluctuations

Less common but still mentioned with some frequency are the following:
- physical exertion
- sexual activity
- changes in the weather
- exposure to glare or bright light
- odors
- high altitude

Trigger conditions may interact with each other. For example, a food trigger may elicit a headache only for some premenstrual women. Psychological stress may trigger a headache only when you are fatigued or have consumed alcohol. If you've had headaches for a long time that are set off by certain triggers, you probably have already learned to avoid them. See table 3.1 in chapter 3 for a list of some the more common triggers.

Many life stressors that may act as headache triggers are more difficult to recognize than food or odor sensitivities. A tension headache arising while you're trying to meet a deadline, or after an argument or a near accident, is more obvious to pinpoint. More subtle, however, is the chronic stress associated with bad jobs, ongoing financial worries, or difficult interpersonal relationships. In the face of such chronic stressors we may experience an underlying sense of depression or anxiety, but these chronic stressors and the resulting mood states can't usually be linked to a specific headache. Rather, chronic stress simply may be associated with a generalized increased tendency to have headaches.

Many times headaches appear out of the blue without an obvious or even a subtle trigger. Such unpredictably is one reason why headaches can be so puzzling and frustrating. It can become difficult to make work commitments, or even plans for an evening, let alone long-range plans. It is at this point that the headache pain, along with the disruption it causes, can be classified as a major life stressor itself. However, if we really work at it, we can usually find some specific

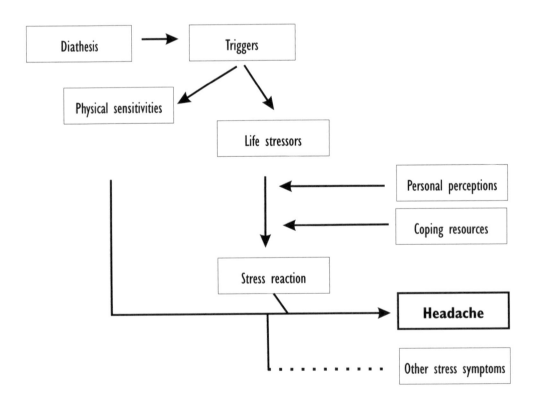

Figure 2.2:   Further Interactions between Headaches and Stressors

headache triggers, be they physical or emotional, or at least learn to recognize some feature in our daily life that may be contributing to an increase in headaches. Figure 2.2 shows the headache model from chapter 1 with further interactions.

It now includes the physiological predisposition (diathesis) to develop headaches. It also includes the fact that the diathesis interacts with triggers. The model now accounts for the fact that not everyone gets headaches, no matter how much life stress they experience, and not everyone with headaches has elevated life stressors. To have headaches you must have both the diathesis and some type of trigger. For some individuals, physical sensitivities are major triggers; for others, life stressors are crucial. Or, it may be a combination of the two. The fact that physical sensitivities may interact with reactions to life stressors is represented by the converging lines leading to "Headache" in figure 2.2.

The Physiology of the Headache

Once a person with a headache diathesis encounters a headache trigger, a complex set of cascading physiological events is set into motion, involving the muscles and the release of neurochemicals that affect blood vessels and nerves. The headache itself is a highly complex physiological event. The goal of all headache therapies, from drugs to self-regulation, is to prevent, stop, or smooth out this chain of pain-producing events.

To understand a headache (or any other type of pain) it is necessary to remember that pain signals from everywhere in the body are interpreted in designated areas of the brain referred to as the *sensory cortex*. The neural transmission route from the source of the pain, through the central nervous system, to the sensory cortex is always convoluted—this allows other parts of the brain to increase or decrease the intensity of the felt pain signal. The ability of the central nervous system to turn incoming pain signals up or down is a physiological principle essential to learning self-regulation.

Emotional/Behavioral Reactions to Headaches

It's very hard to be totally indifferent to a severe headache, especially one that has the habit of returning. With the initial signs of a pending migraine attack, or even with the first tinge of muscle tension pain, alarming thoughts and feelings surface like, "Oh no not again; I don't have time for a headache today; I just can't stand to go through this again!" The headache episode can result in a terrible feeling of being trapped, with anxious desperation over how you're going to manage your life that day. If this happens often enough, frustration, anger, and depression are almost inevitable. Thus, the headache, which may be a response to stressors, perpetuates the vicious cycle and becomes a stressor itself.

Think about how a headache can sometimes make you feel embarrassed, guilty, or angry about retreating from your responsibilities. Family and co-workers, even when understanding, may have a hard time not becoming irritated with you. Some people with headaches report an internal feeling of emotional agitation tied to the sheer inconvenience of it all. Unfortunately, such negative reactions can amplify the pain signals in the brain to an even higher pitch. Your mood while in the throes of a headache can work like the volume dial on a radio or TV. Neural networks in the brain that transfer signals to the sensory cortex actually do function somewhat like an electronic amplifier. Therefore, remaining calm and relaxed, although very difficult while in pain, can be one aspect of controlling the pain sensation itself.

In summary, a psychophysiological analysis of headaches includes the following components:

1. A *diathesis*—or a physical predisposition for nerves, muscles, and blood vessels to produce headaches.

2. A sensitivity to *trigger* mechanisms, sometimes obvious, but often subtle, that sets off the headache in someone with a physiological diathesis. In some cases, the triggers may never be clearly identified.

3. The *headache* pain itself, resulting from a cascade of physical events that led to the pain, set off by the headache trigger.

4. The thoughts, feelings, and behaviors that constitute our cognitive and emotional *reactions* to the headache, which can amplify the pain or turn it down.

Classification and Mechanisms of Headache Types

What exactly makes up the above-mentioned cascade of physiological events leading to a headache? Only ten or fifteen years ago researchers were quite sure that most benign headache pain came from either tight muscles of the head and neck (muscle tension headache), or dilated blood vessels (vascular headache), or a combination of muscular and vascular effects (mixed headache). However, recent studies indicate that this simple dichotomy is an oversimplification (Hatch 1992; Olsen 1991). Even when muscle and blood vessel peculiarities are found with headaches, it is no longer clear whether these are the only, or even the primary, sources of pain.

Tension Headaches

It is estimated that at least 50 percent of the population suffers at least occasionally from tension headaches. In fact, tension headaches may be the most common pain disorder of our contemporary age, possibly as a symptom of the stress of modern life.

You may be confused by the multiple meanings of the word "tension." Sometimes the word implies the emotional arousal caused by the hassles of daily life. Other times, the term is used to refer specifically to the mechanical contraction of muscles in the head and neck that bring on a tension headache. In the latter case, the terms "tension" and "muscular contraction" or "musculoskeletal" headache are used synonymously. But because it is no longer certain that muscle tension is actually the primary source of pain in a tension headache, you might be better off to think of a tension headache simply as a particular pattern of symptoms, regardless of their source.

As a rule, tension headaches include most of the following characteristics:

1. The pain is gradual in onset, often beginning in the upper neck and back of the head and working forward.

2. The pain is highly variable in intensity and duration from one headache episode to another.

3. The pain is experienced as a "band" of tightness, heaviness, or pressure around the head.

4. The pain is constant rather than throbbing, but it may wax and wane over the course of a day.

5. The pain is bilateral (affecting both sides of the head).

6. The pain often becomes worse over the course of the day, especially on busy, stress-filled days.

For some people excessive tension, and sometimes spasms, of the powerful muscles controlling the jaw often play a role in chronic tension headaches. Jaw tension may be emotional in origin, but can also be caused by poor tooth alignment and other dental problems.

Muscle dysfunction can come from several sources in addition to the jaw. First, tight muscles in the shoulders, neck, and head become fatigued and irritated. Just imagine how painful your hand would become if you clenched your fist hour after hour. Tightness of the muscles in the head and neck can have a similar effect. Second, blood flow to tight muscles can be pinched off, causing the muscles to suffer from an inadequate blood supply, adding to the pain. Third, tensed muscles can put pressure on nerves and blood vessels, pinching them between the skull and the surrounding bands of muscle fibers, causing a secondary source of pain. This secondary pain can feel like a burning, throbbing, neuralgic irritation, combined with the characteristic dull ache of the tension headache. In some cases, a tension headache may trigger the even more severe pain of a vascular headache.

At the heart of the current confusion regarding the exact role of muscle tension are studies that fail to reliably find elevated muscle tension, or other muscle abnormality, in those experiencing tension headaches. It is now believed that even though muscle tightness or spasm sometimes may be directly related to such headaches, it is primarily the neurochemical agitation of the nerve endings in the course of the muscle activity that directly corresponds to the pain. Once sensory nerves are stirred up by the release of certain pain-producing neuroactive biochemicals, relaxing the involved muscles alone is not going to relieve the pain immediately. This interpretation is supported by evidence that tension headache patients often exhibit increased tenderness and lowered pain pressure thresholds (Hatch 1992; Langemark 1989; Lous and Olsen 1982). With nerve endings highly sensitized to any pressure, even normal amounts of muscle activation can become pain producing.

Migraine Headaches

Migraine headaches are the best known of the vascular headaches—those headaches that arise from changes in blood vessels in the face, head, and neck. These blood vessels are sometimes unnaturally narrowed (vasoconstriction), usually followed by a rebound period of unnatural widening (vasodilation).

Vascular headaches are less common than tension headaches, affecting approximately 20 percent of adults. Two-thirds of these adults are female, a fact that suggests a possible hormonal link. Most migraine headaches are felt on one side of the head, and are commonly associated with a particular blood vessel in the temple, or above or behind one of the eyes. The definition of the term "migraine" itself is "pain on one side of the head." It is a pain that can't be ignored. Migraine sufferers often become very sensitive to light when one of these headaches strikes and the pain can be so intense that it overwhelms their ability to attend to even routine activities. The chronic migraine sufferer will almost always seek medical help eventually.

A migraine is the outcome of a complex process involving the neurologic and neurochemical regulation of blood vessels in the head and neck. What triggers this process of constriction and dilation is not clear. It is thought that brain-regulating hormones originating in the hypothalamus may alter the level of circulating neurotransmitters such as serotonin and norepinpherine, which, in turn, affects the nerves that control the volume of blood flow through the arteries of the scalp and brain. It is known that circulating serotonin is high in the brain just before a migraine starts but low during the headache itself. Emotional stress or excitement may start this entire process, although emotional stress is not the only trigger. Hormonal changes, temperature changes, and food, drink, and drug reactions are also common triggers.

Whatever the trigger, the somatic process appears to begin with vasoconstriction, causing localized obstruction of the blood supply in the brain, which appears to be responsible for the initial warning aura (changes in vision, tingling or weakness of the limbs, dizziness, or faintness), which signals an impending migraine attack. The vasoconstriction then stimulates the production of the counterregulatory neurochemicals that maintain adequate blood flow (and thus proper nutrition) in the brain cells. When this corrective effort is too vigorous and overshoots the normal target level, it produces a "rebound" vasodilation. This excessive dilation and the subsequent swelling of certain blood vessels, which corresponds to the throbbing, painful stage of the migraine, is thought to irritate nerve endings in the walls of the overstretched blood vessels.

The direct relationship between arterial blood flow in swollen arteries and migraine headaches also has been challenged by recent research. At this point, we can best say that the correspondence between the level of blood flow in the affected area of the head and the level of pain is very fuzzy. Here again, the status of nerve endings bathed in pain-generating biochemicals is probably the key to the pain. Blood flow changes associated with sharp changes in vasoconstriction and vasodilation certainly remain part of the picture, but seemingly they aren't the whole picture.

Migraine with Aura

The classic migraine, with aura, usually includes the following characteristics:

1. The pain is preceded by initial warning signs, called an *aura*. See figure 2.3.

   a. Changes in vision are the most common signs: blind spots, zigzag lines (so-called fortification schemata), flashing lights, and tunnel vision

   b. Feelings of dizziness, faintness, and weakness

   c. Mood changes: depression, irritability, and restlessness

2. The pain is unilateral (on one side of the head), often focused in one temple, or above or behind one eye. That eye and the nose on the affected side may become runny.

3. The pain is often accompanied by nausea and vomiting, a so-called "sick" headache.

4. The pain can sometimes be prevented with vasoconstricting drugs.

5. This headache pattern is often found in close relatives, which suggests an inherited predisposition.

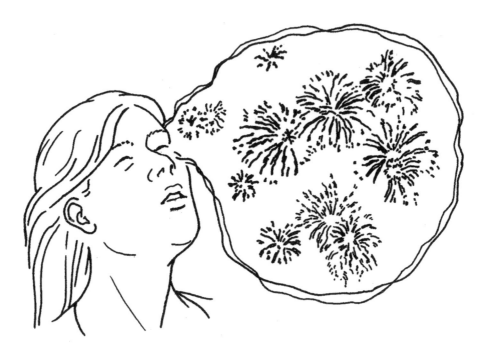

Figure 2.3:   **Flashing Lights**

Migraine without Aura

Actually, only about 15 percent of migraine headaches fit the above-described classic pattern of *migraine with aura*. More frequent are vascular headaches that lack the distinctive initial aura, which warns of an oncoming migraine, and that may not be distinctively unilateral in nature. This more common pattern, formerly referred to as a "common" migraine, is now simply called *migraine without aura*. People who experience a nearly constant painful daily headache are likely to have either this type of headache or a variation of the mixed headache described below.

Mixed Headache

We now recognize that many chronic headache sufferers experience symptoms of both tension and vascular headaches. This pattern, called a *mixed headache*, has symptoms characteristic of either headache type. The two types of symptoms may occur simultaneously or sequentially, although usually the muscle tension will be noticeable at first. Typically though, the more intense vascular symptoms will prompt a person to see a doctor.

Doctor Bakal, who was previously described as one of the chief proponents of a psychobiological view of headaches, has provided considerable research evidence indicating that there is a high degree of overlap of muscle contraction with migraine headaches symptoms. He argues that most headache sufferers experience some symptoms of both musculoskeletal and vascular headaches. As the headaches become increasingly severe, however, the vascular symptoms become more dominant. Furthermore, he states that the overlap of symptoms argues against the theory that migraine headaches are genetic in origin while tension headaches are acquired. Both types may involve genetic factors and the emergence of a psychobiological predisposition (Bakal 1994).

Cluster Headaches

Still another vascular headache pattern is the so-called *cluster headache*. These are intense vascular headaches that are usually brief in duration (often about twenty minutes). They have been given the name "cluster" because they can occur with great frequency over a period of several hours, days, or weeks, and will then disappear for several months before returning again. Although brief in duration, these headaches can produce the most severe pain of all chronic benign headache syndromes. Tearing eyes and a sweating forehead on the side of the head where the pain is located are common. Cluster headaches are quite rare and are experienced by more men than woman. The mechanisms are very poorly understood and they can be very difficult to treat.

Sinus Headaches

Sinus headaches are mentioned here because they are often confused with migraines. The sinuses are air pockets within the bones of the nose, cheeks, and forehead. Mucous secreted in the linings of these air pockets normally drains through the nose. Oversecretion, blockage, or infection can increase sinus pressure and cause pain that is felt across the cheeks and forehead. Sinus headaches often respond to treatment with decongestants and mild, painkilling medications. Severe headaches in the region of the sinuses, in the absence of sinus congestion, actually may be vascular headaches involving blood vessels in or near the sinuses.

Some headache experts believe that most "sinus headaches" are an invention of commercial advertisers pushing endless sinus headache remedies. It's possible that many of the so-called sinus headaches are not truly linked to sinus congestion at all, but are actually seasonal variations of migraines or other vascular headaches.

Posttraumatic Headaches

Posttraumatic headaches following a head and/or neck injury often are accompanied by several of the following symptoms:

1. Head may ache at site of injury, but discomfort also may be generalized to entire head and neck

2. Fatigability (becoming easily tired or exhausted) and need for extra sleep

3. Dizziness and blurred vision

4. Problems with memory, attention, and concentration

5. Feeling confused and disoriented

6. Depression and anxiety

Both muscle tension and migraine symptoms may follow a head or neck injury. These symptoms are common for a day or two after a head injury, but the pain usually resolves in a week or two. However, in some cases, even with a minor injury showing no other signs of brain damage, headaches may persist, possibly because of difficulties with muscles that may have been damaged. The severity of the chronic headache may be unrelated to the severity of the head injury. Often it's accompanied by difficulty in paying attention and concentrating, and in mood alterations.

Whenever minor head and/or neck trauma seem to trigger unrelenting headaches, patients and doctors alike can quickly become frustrated. Suspicion that the reports of pain are exaggerated is all too frequent with so-called "whiplash" injury. When nothing shows up "broken" on Xrays following such accidents, it's easy to overlook the possibility of painful overextension injuries to muscles and nerves and blood vessels of the back and neck. Sometimes, neuropsychological testing for subtle indicators of head injury can be revealing. If pain continues for more than a few days, it is particularly important that these patients not simply be given medication; they also must receive the type of physical therapy evaluation described in chapter 6.

Headaches can, of course, result from severe injuries to the neck or head. However, discussion of injury to brain and spinal cord structures is well beyond the scope of this book. Self-regulation strategies are certainly important adjuncts for managing pain stemming from such injuries, although we are no longer dealing with benign conditions in such cases.

Rebound Headaches

The concept of *rebound* is very important to understanding headaches and the rationale behind various treatments. Any of the above-described headaches can occur in the form of a rebound headache. So, the rebound headache is not a unique form of headache; rather, its uniqueness lies in the circumstances in which it appears.

The physiological concept of rebound stems from the notion that anything that activates the body in one direction potentially can set the stage for the opposite reaction. For example, if the nervous system is calmed by tranquilizing medication for a prolonged period of time, abrupt discontinuation of the tranquilizers will result in the opposite effect—agitation and tension. Likewise, abrupt withdrawal of narcotic painkillers frequently causes rebound pain.

The drug caffeine illustrates some of the complications of rebound effects. Caffeine is a vasoconstrictor—it shrinks blood vessels. Small amounts of caffeine taken occasionally, whether in the form of coffee, colas, or medications, can help control headaches associated with vasodilation. But it can also become part of a rebound pattern, as some of you may have noticed if you go without your morning coffee. The irony of caffeine use is that even though it can relieve a headache, excessive use also can contribute to headaches thanks to the rebound effect. For some heavy coffee drinkers, anytime the blood level of caffeine drops, the full-blown rebound headache may return.

The concept of rebound is not limited to drug effects. It also applies to natural events occurring within the body because of the physiological process of *homeostasis* (internal physiological balance). Internal homeostatic rebound may be the key to understanding another perplexing experience of many headache sufferers. This is the so-called *weekend*, *relaxation*, or *vacation* headache. Many migraine sufferers with rebound features are convinced that their headaches have absolutely nothing to do with stress, because their worse headaches do not occur at busy times or under the stress of deadlines. In fact, the pattern seems to be just the opposite; headaches strike only after the task has been completed and the person is ready to relax. Some students know all too well the routine of getting a headache only when final exams are over and it's time to take some rest and recreation. Thus, it seems the triggers are things like sleeping, a quiet weekend, or an extended vacation.

The key to understanding this paradoxical poststress headache onset lies in recognizing its rebound nature. For those with this headache pattern, the physiological reactions to stressors don't cause head pain directly; instead they set the stage for the future headache. The preheadache stress phase may result in increased release of a number of stress neurohormones that may stimulate sympathetic activation. The sympathetic activation, in turn, may stimulate vasoconstriction of sensitive blood vessels in the migraine-prone person. In the tension headache-prone person, the sympathetic activation may lead to the release of neurochemicals that eventually cause nerve endings in the head and neck to become highly pressure-sensitive. Because the body is always trying to maintain internal homeostasis, this increase in neurohormonal activation activity also stimulates counterregulatory neurohormonal activity. Once the stressor event is over and you have the opportunity to relax, this counterregulatory effort may be so powerful that it overshoots the mark, causing the opposite vascular response, namely, overdilation. Unfortunately, along with the swelling of the overdilated artery comes the ironic "relaxation" headache.

The stress reaction described above is often referred to as the "fight-or-flight response," which is discussed in more detail in chapter 4. The rebound occurs with the turning off of this stress reaction. Both drugs and self-regulation training can address smoothing out the internal physiological rebound that leads to headaches. This is a very important concept for you to understand and remember as we proceed into the treatment of headaches.

Key Word Summary

To ensure that you have thoroughly mastered the material in this chapter, write the definition of each term below in your own words. Future chapters will build on your understanding of these terms.

Trigger: _____

_____

_____

Diathesis: _____

_____

_____

Tension headache: _____

_____

_____

Migraine headache: _____

_____

_____

Prodrome: _____

_____

_____

Posttraumatic headache: _____

_____

_____

Rebound: _____

_____

_____

Further Reading

Diamond, S. D. and D. J. Dalessio. 1992. *The Practicing Physician's Approach to Headache.* 5th ed. Baltimore: Williams & Wilkins.

Edeling, J. 1988. *Manual Therapy for Chronic Headache.* London: Butterworths & Co. Ltd.

Spierings, E.L.H. 1996. *Management of Migraine.* Boston: Butterworth-Heinemann.

CHAPTER 3

A Plan For Coping

▲ What "control" of headaches means

▲ What to do to control your headaches

▲ Possible headache triggers

▲ Specific headache triggers

It is important to have a plan for dealing with your headaches. Having a sense of what you can do will in itself make the headache more tolerable and help you to overcome the feeling that you're a helpless victim of a force totally out of your control.

What "Control" of Headaches Means

Throughout this book there is an emphasis on the importance of you feeling in control of your headaches, rather than feeling that the headaches control you. Nothing is worse than feeling intolerable pain with no particular plan for dealing with it—it is truly like riding a "runaway freight train." In such cases, the *fear* of headaches can become part of a chronic stress pattern that makes the headache experience even worse. When the fear of headaches leads to more headaches, you really are trapped in a quagmire.

If you can't make social commitments for an evening, can't go to a store or restaurant, or can't plan a vacation because you are afraid you couldn't cope if you were to get a headache, then your headaches are in control. Similarly, if you are missing too many work days, can't advance in your career, or risk losing your job because of headaches—your headaches are in control. In short, if the course of events in your life has been altered by headaches, they are controlling you.

Part of being in control is having a plan worked out with your doctor. If you frequently go to a hospital emergency room, or randomly take any medication you can lay your hands on, that indicates you have an inadequate management plan. Emergency room care is a very ineffective and potentially dangerous way to deal with a nonemergency pain condition. Emergency room physicians can't be expected to understand your unique headache pattern, or how your other medical problems or treatments may be contributing to your headaches. Neither are they in a position to monitor carefully whether their prescriptions are actually contributing to your headache cycle. Finally, an emergency room is not a place where you can expect to get a multidisciplinary view on headache management.

Feeling in control doesn't mean that you will never have another headache. What it does mean, first and foremost, is having the confidence that there are things you can do to:

1. Prevent or reduce the frequency of headaches

2. Reduce the severity if one begins

3. Make it through the occasional full-blown headache without feeling overwhelmed.

A second and broader meaning of feeling in control is having the confidence that headache pain, although it may be an inconvenience, won't dictate the events of your daily life.

A Rating Scale for Headache Pain

0   *No pain*

1–2   *Slight pain:* I am aware of it only when I think about it

3–4   *Mild pain:* I can ignore it most of the time

5–6   *Moderate pain:* cannot be ignored, but I can still continue with all my normal activities

7–8   *Severe pain:* makes concentration difficult, but I can still manage tasks that are not too difficult

9–10 *Intense, incapacitating pain:* nearly impossible for me to do anything with this much pain

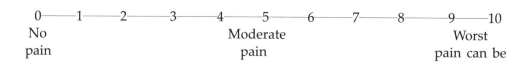

Pain is always a subjective phenomenon, such that we can never be entirely sure what someone else is feeling. Nevertheless, it can be useful to have some numbers to use as reference points when talking to your doctor, or for keeping a headache record. Researchers find a surprising degree of similarity from person to person in how a scale from 0 to 10 is used—where 0 is no pain and 10 is the worst pain possible. A 1 or 2 is almost always described as slight discomfort. Most people also agree that a pain below 5 or 6 may be a nuisance but can usually be ignored, and they still can go on with normal routines. At 8, pain becomes a major challenge and at the level of 9 or 10 the pain interferes with attention and concentration to such a degree it is impossible to carry on normal activity. (More detailed headache rating logs are provided in chapter 5.)

Ideally, being in control means keeping headaches away from the critical 8, 9, or 10 range. But, sometimes, it may mean knowing only that you can wait out a bad level 10 headache for a few hours because you know it will be better tomorrow. Even better is to know that once a headache starts you can do something, including taking a pill, retiring to a quiet, dark room, or doing self-relaxation exercises that will keep the pain at an 8 or lower. Thus, control applies to all three aspects of headache control—*prevention* of headache, *reduction* of severity, and *tolerance* when necessary.

Daily Stress Log

Just as it is useful to rate your headache discomfort on a regular basis, it can also be useful to rate your cognitive and physical signs of stress. These ratings can help you to become aware of your reactions to stressors and to begin to think about their possible relationships to your headaches.

Each person's typical response to stressors is unique. In the sample below, the headache sufferer lists two cognitive and three physiological indicators of stress, and rates each indicator four times a day. Imagine that this person spent the morning with some mild signs of stress as he or she anticipated an important afternoon meeting with a supervisor. The meeting was indeed difficult and the signs of stress were very high, but they tapered off over the evening and caused little sleep difficulty at night. Sleep was rated only once because it applied only during "nighttime" hours. Note which stress indicator was clearly the most situationally specific response for this person.

Daily Stress Log Sample

Stress Indicator	Morning	Afternoon	Evening	Nighttime
Can't concentrate	4	6	3	0
Poor sleep				0
Tightness in throat	5	8	4	1
Cold/damp hands	2	9	2	0
Gastrointestinal stress	3	5	4	1

Stress Severity Scale

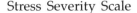
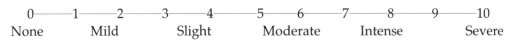

0———1———2———3———4———5———6———7———8———9———10
None   Mild   Slight   Moderate   Intense   Severe

Now, fill in this blank log to get a sense of your daily stressors and how they correspond to your headaches.

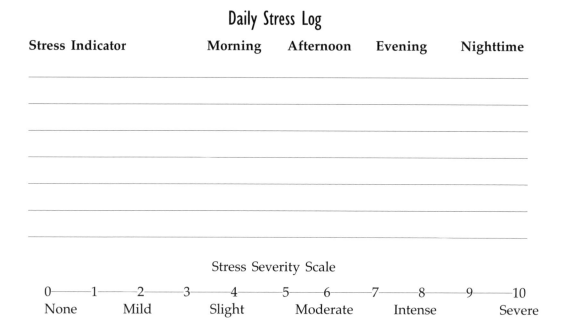

Daily Stress Log

Stress Indicator	Morning	Afternoon	Evening	Nighttime

Stress Severity Scale

0——1——2——3——4——5——6——7——8——9——10
None   Mild   Slight   Moderate   Intense   Severe

What You Can Do to Increase Your Control

1. Recognize Your Headache Triggers
   The first thing to do on your own is to learn about and try to control your exposure to what may be your headache triggers. Avoiding any food or drink that can trigger a headache is obvious. If you are sensitive to cigarette smoke, cosmetics, perfumes, or the odor of cleaning fluids, it may take some work to avoid them. You might have to be assertive enough to politely request that a relative, friend, or co-worker not use those products in your presence. Some triggers can be very hard to circumvent; for example, you can't completely avoid weather changes. But you can think ahead—if heat or cold seem to be triggers, try to be prepared by wearing the most adaptive clothing. Carry a hat to keep your head warm in the winter and another to keep it cool in the summer. If excessive fatigue, sleeping irregular hours, or sleeping late on weekends set off headaches, work on improving your sleep habits. See table 3.1. Take into account more indirect triggers as well, for instance, a lack of exercise will seldom appear as a direct trigger of headaches, but generally poor physical fitness leaves you more vulnerable to stress effects. Sometimes, little things make a big difference between feeling you have some control over your headaches or that they are controlling you. Many common triggers in food and drink are listed in table 3.2.

   When thinking about avoiding headache triggers, don't forget about *interacting* triggers. Are you sensitive to certain foods or scents only when fatigued, at a certain time in your hormonal cycle, after an illness, or while feeling stressed? Remain alert, but try not to worry so much about triggers that your vigilance becomes yet another source of stress. Find the balance that works for you. Stories are told about people who eat nothing but a few selected dried fruits and grains and never leave their air-conditioned homes for fear of a headache. Unfortunately, in such cases avoidance of the headache becomes as much of an activity-restricting handicap as the headache itself.

2. Learn to Use Over-the-Counter Medications
   By all means use over-the-counter medications such as aspirin or ibuprofen if they help control your headaches. But remain sensitive to the fact that these and all over-the-counter medications can cause problems if used excessively. Stomach upset is particularly common with aspirin. Also, if you are on medications for other conditions, be aware of possible harmful drug interactions. This topic is addressed in detail in chapter 8.

3. Appraise the Role Your Lifestyle Plays in Your Headaches
   Be open and honest with yourself. If drinking alcohol is contributing to your headaches, are you willing to deal with this problem? The same is true for diet and exercise. Although overall good health and fitness certainly don't guarantee a headache-free life, they can help.
   What about stress? Some highly productive individuals simply take on too much. If this is true of you, why do you do so? Is it really necessary or do you need to feel indispensable? Do you face stressors that you can reduce or eliminate? Make a list of the stressors in your life that can and cannot be controlled. Try to change those that fall into the first category. And for those in the latter category, learn to reduce their impact on your body via self-regulation techniques.

4. Learn and Practice Self-Regulation Techniques
   Self-regulating techniques, the primary focus of this book, will help you gain a sense of control over your headaches. Although the term self-regulation is used most often to refer to cognitive mental focusing for altering physical systems, it can also be thought of more broadly to include anything and everything you can do for your headaches. Thus, monitoring your headache triggers, adjusting your lifestyle, improving your physical fitness, even finding a doctor with whom you can effectively communicate can all be considered part of a self-regulation strategy.

5. Develop a Philosophical Attitude
   We often joke about the fact that the only sure things in life are death and taxes. Maybe we should add pain to our list of sure things. Every living person must come to grips with the fact that not only death, but injury, illness, and pain strike indiscriminately. Often there is no answer to "Why me?" Sometimes, doctors can't even tell us the source of our pain. Effective treatments may be partial at best. You may feel it's unfair that you or a loved one should have to suffer this way. You are absolutely right: usually it is unfair. However, life comes with no guarantees of fairness. And there is something you can do about your headaches—practice self-regulation techniques.

Table 3.1: Factors That May Contribute to Headaches

Table 3.1 provides a list of factors that might trigger headaches or contribute to an increase in headaches. Check off (✓) all those that could apply to you, and double-check (✓✓) those that you believe are likely to relate to your headaches. Consider which factors you can do something about.

	Today	Past Month	Past Year
Foods with (see table 3.2)			
• tyramine _____			
• sodium nitrate or nitrite _____			
• monosodium glutamate _____			
• phenylethylamine _____			
Drinks with			
• alcohol _____			
• caffeine _____			
Airborne Exposure to			
• too much dust or mold _____			
• indoor smoke and fumes _____			
• outdoor air pollution _____			
• cosmetics: e.g., perfume _____			
Medications			
• increasing use of _____			
• analgesics _____			
• changes in medications _____			
Behaviors			
• not enough sleep _____			
• too much sleeping _____			
• poor quality of sleep _____			
• poor diet, overeating _____			
• or skipping meals _____			
• no time for recreation _____			
• or relaxation _____			
• smoking _____			
• not enough exercise _____			

Table 3.1: Factors That May Contribute to Headaches (continued)

	Today	Past Month	Past Year
General Health			
• indigestion			
• asthma			
• diabetes			
• high blood pressure			
• low blood pressure			
• back pain			
• other chronic condition			
• recent injury			
• dizziness, lightheadedness			
• chest pain			
• other health			
Women Only			
• irregular periods			
• PMS			
• period started (hormonal)			
• menopause symptoms			
• other ob/gyn			
Cognitive/Mood			
• frustrated			
• angry			
• depressed			
• guilty			
• anxious			
• feel tense/restless			
• can't concentrate			
• mind racing			
Physical—Breathing			
• hyperventilation (rapid, shallow breath)			
• holding breath			
• can't get enough air			

Table 3.1: Factors That May Contribute to Headaches (continued)

	Today	Past Month	Past Year
Physical—Muscles			
• clenching teeth			
• neck/upper back tight			
• frowning, facial grimace			
• poor posture			
• head and neck			
• remainder of body			
Physical—Autonomic/Endocrine			
• cold hands			
• excessive nervous sweating			
• rapid heart beat			
• stomach/throat feel tight			
• chest pain			
Stressors—Situational			
• financial			
• job concerns			
• marriage			
• sex			
• children			
• other social relations			
• other:			
Stressors—Personal			
• lonely or isolated			
• low self-esteem			
• too perfectionistic			
• low self-confidence			
• too impatient			
• other:			

If you must spend a few hours in a dark, quiet room with ice or heat applied to your head and/or neck, can you do so without feeling trapped, overwhelmed, or angry? Can you say calmly to yourself, "Some days a headache is just part of my life"?

Table 3.2: Triggering Ingredients and Common Sources

Listed below are some of the most common foods and drinks containing chemicals that can cause dilation or constriction of blood vessels and thereby trigger migraine headaches.

Amines: Tyramine and Phenylethylamine
- found in anything that is smoked, pickled, or fermented
- aged cheese, chocolate, red wine, nuts, smoked fish, pickled food, sour cream, chicken liver, broad beans, fresh yeast breads

Sodium Nitrates and Nitrites
- commonly found in processed meats
- ham, sausage, bologna, hot dogs, luncheon meats, bacon, cured fish

Monosodium Glutamate
- commercial seasonings and preservatives
- many Chinese foods, many canned and frozen foods
- alcohol
- all forms of alcohol especially red wine, brandy, and gin

Caffeine
- coffee, tea, soft drinks, chocolate
- many over-the-counter analgesics and stimulants

Getting Medical Help

If your headaches are infrequent, measure 5 or less on our 0–10-point rating scale, and can be controlled by whatever you can do on your own, you need do little more. But if sufficient control does not result from those efforts, it's time to create a plan with a doctor.

People vary a great deal in how quickly they bring a pain symptom to a doctor, including headaches. There is no simple guideline other than common sense. If you had a parent or close relative who had headaches and died prematurely of a tumor or stroke, common sense for you might be to seek medical reassurance that your headache is not indicative of a dangerous underlying condition. Even with minor headaches, it is a good idea to mention them to your primary care physician during the course of a routine physical exam. And, as mentioned before, anytime you might have an exceptionally severe headache—unlike anything you have ever experienced before—it should be reported to your doctor immediately. If such a headache is accompanied by changes in vision, sensation, weakness, or state of mental alertness, it may be a medical emergency.

Your doctor should be willing to work with you on a plan for your headaches, even if they are only minor. The plan may be a simple one. For example, you might be given a list of possible headache triggers and instructed to keep a diary of your headaches to help you spot any possible sensitivities. Your doctor will also help you decide at what point to use medication, both over-the-counter and prescription drugs.

A doctor who seems too quick to give out potent painkillers, especially narcotics, accompanied by vague instructions to "use as needed," hasn't put enough work into your treatment plan. It's exactly this type of vague treatment that has gotten far too many patients into trouble both with increasing pain and increasing medication dependency.

Referral to a Headache Specialist

There are differences of opinion about when a referral should be made to a headache specialist, usually a neurologist. As a rule, it is preferable to let your primary care physician decide—it's expensive and not very helpful to overtest, overdiagnose, and overtreat routine headaches, and most primary care doctors will recognize the difference quickly. But if you feel a referral is needed, don't hesitate to raise the point, especially if your doctor seems indifferent, has no plan, or, after an adequate trial, the plan is clearly not helping. Unfortunately, there are doctors who are just not very interested in dealing with benign headaches.

A specialist will usually establish the diagnosis of the type of headache you have and if indicated, order more tests. Don't insist on more tests such as MRIs if the specialist (based on a thorough office exam) doesn't feel this is needed. As with a primary care doctor, if the specialist seems unsympathetic and uninterested in developing a plan with you, you have a right to ask for a second opinion.

Developing a Management Plan with Your Doctor

A good plan is whatever helps you feel that your headaches are under your control. A good treatment plan worked out with your doctor should include the following components:

1. A careful review of sensitivities that may trigger headaches and a willingness to discuss and review the topic of headache triggers.

2. Attention to other health issues. Perhaps your headaches are related to medication you're currently taking for some other condition? How about birth control pills or other hormones? How is your general health and overall physical fitness? If exertion brings on a headache, is it because you have an underlying cardiovascular problem, or is it that you simply have very poor aerobic fitness? As will be stressed in later chapters, mus-

cular functioning and posture problems involving the head, neck, and back are often overlooked in contributing to headaches. Has your doctor considered a physical therapy evaluation?

3. A plan for what, when, and how to use medication. When it comes to managing headaches, medications can be your greatest friend or worst enemy. You and your doctor must appreciate the difference. This is an area where a doctor must pay close attention to what you say about a medication's effects, and be knowledgeable and ready with a range of options.

   Different types of headaches, differing in frequency and severity, and following different courses over time usually require quite different drug treatment. Normally, occasional headaches will call for medications to relieve symptoms. Frequent and severe headaches will require preventive medications as well as medications to alleviate symptoms. You must have a medication plan that you understand and that doesn't leave you with intolerable side effects. What else you expect to be able to do while having a headache should be taken into consideration. Will you be at home or at work? Will you need to drive? Chapter 8 provides details regarding specific medications and medication plans.

4. Pay attention to your lifestyle, your personality and coping skills, and daily life circumstances. Most doctors specializing in headaches are aware of the relationship between stress and headaches. Even so, many will ignore the issue because they don't feel qualified dealing with psycho-physiological matters. Don't act insulted when your doctor brings up lifestyle issues or asks you to consider consultation with a stress-management therapist. This doesn't mean that your doctor believes your headache pain is not really serious, nor does it necessarily mean that he or she feels you are using too much medication. Usually, it means that the doctor, based on experience, feels that a treatment plan that includes learning self-regulation skills will have a more successful outcome.

Your Right to Ask for Treatment Options

Both primary care doctors and headache specialists should be willing to honor a headache patient's request for evaluation and possible treatment by alternative therapists for such options as physical therapy, massage, biofeedback, or other stress-management therapies. Many will be happy to do so, sometimes being pleasantly surprised to find a patient eager to explore options other than medication. A few doctors may object on the grounds that such options are too expensive for routine headaches. However, in light of the mounting evidence that these are safe and helpful techniques, I believe such an attitude is very short-sighted. A younger patient who learns that exercise and self-regulation routines can help with a troubling headache syndrome may have dramatically reduced lifetime medical costs. Conversely, once headaches escalate and lead to frequent emergency room visits, endless trials of medication, and repeated neuro-imaging tests, the cumulative costs will mount rapidly.

Key Word Summary

To ensure that you have thoroughly mastered the material in this chapter, write the definition of each term below in your own words. Future chapters will build on your understanding of these terms.

Indirect triggers: _____

_____

_____

Stress indicator: _____

_____

_____

Interacting triggers: _____

_____

_____

Lifestyle (role of): _____

_____

_____

Stress-management therapies: _____

_____

_____

_____

_____

Further Reading

Cady, R. and K. Farmer. 1993. *Headache Free*. New York: Bantam Books.

Diamond, S. and D. J. Dalessio. 1982. *The Practicing Physician's Approach to Headache*. 3rd ed. Baltimore: William & Wilkins.

Saper, J. R. and K. R. Magee. 1981. *Freedom From Headaches*. New York: Simon & Schuster.

Rapoport, A. M. and F. D. Sheftell. 1990. *Headache Relief*. New York: Simon & Schuster.

CHAPTER 4

Steps to Taking Control

▲ The fight-or-flight response

▲ Self-regulation

▲ The building blocks

▲ Self-monitoring

▲ Self-regulating scripts

Section I: The Building Blocks of Self-Regulation

This chapter explains the neurophysiological foundation for using focused attention for slow-deep breathing, muscle relaxation, hand warming, and mental imagery as the building blocks of self-regulation. As you increase your understanding of your own physiology, you can begin using the self-regulating techniques provided in this chapter. When you realize how your mind and body work together, self-regulation will feel like a very natural activity.

Pain Is Felt in the Brain

Remember, all sensations are felt only when nerve impulses reach the sensory cortex of the brain. It has been recognized for thousands of years that because pain is experienced in the brain, it can be modulated by psychological states, such as attention and emotion. For example, it is well-known that people can perform heroic feats of strength with broken bones, not even realizing they are injured until the event is over. Only recently have we begun to understand how much the nervous system modulates pain sensations.

Neural Circuitry

Think of your brain as a very complex monitoring station that receives information from millions of incoming wires (nerves) and decides what action is taken in response. This is true for all sensory information, whether it be sight, sound, taste, smell, or a somatic sensation. The pain-sensitive nerve endings, running throughout every part of your body, are like a fire alarm ready to send a signal and alert your brain to danger. Sometimes, however, the pain alarm is louder than necessary. It may even be a false alarm. Many headaches are such false alarms. Although some headaches do indicate serious underlying damage, such as tumors or strokes, most of the time pain-sensitive nerve endings in the scalp, face, or neck are just irritated and represent no real danger to the headache sufferer.

Once a pain message reaches the brain, some surprising things can happen. For example, as stated in chapter 3, the brain can adjust the volume of the pain signal. How the pain signal feels partially depends on what else is occupying the brain at the time. In the limbic (emotional) centers of the brain, the pain signal jumps through many kinds of neural circuits that can greatly amplify what is felt. Furthermore, pain-stirred emotions can stir up worries, past painful experiences, and concerns about the personal meaning of the pain. The meaning can intensify the pain further. It seems as if pain, especially if long lasting, finds all the old "tapes" containing all your concerns about job, family, hobbies, sex life, and self-esteem. It can feel as if the pain not only hurts, but also is driving you crazy. Eventually it can become difficult to think straight, relax, or sleep. The pain seems to be in control.

Effects on the Body

When the persistent pain of a headache begins to dominate the neural circuits in our brains, the headache itself becomes a stressor that perpetuates its own vicious cycle. Like any other stressor it can trigger a physical reaction. It can raise our heart rate and blood pressure, and make us clench our teeth, tighten our muscles, and sweat. These physical reactions make us feel worse. This is actually seen in recent brain scan research that shows increased metabolic activity in the sensory cortex as the volunteers anticipate, or actually experience, an experimental pain stimulus (e.g. Drevets, et al., 1995). It may be more than a figure of speech when we encourage patients via self-regulation not to let the pain "use up too much space in your brain."

Many pain-reducing drugs work by turning down the activity in the pain circuits of both the brain and spinal cord. Unfortunately, the result may be that the neural circuits become so slow that the person feels drowsy and sluggish and, occasionally, dizzy and nauseous. Thus, while drugs may temporarily relieve the vicious cycle of pain, and sleep may improve with medication, most people feel their energy is drained by the medication. With the mental and physical calming brought about through self-regulation techniques, we try to turn down the volume of the pain in the nervous system, but in a way that allows the person to feel alert and able to function.

The Fight-or-Flight Response

Was there ever a time when you felt really nervous? Maybe it was just before a presentation you had to give to a group of people, or during a job interview. Try to remember exactly how you felt. What kind of thoughts did you have? Were you able to keep your nervousness in check and see yourself as organized, clear, and confident? Did you breathe comfortably, or did you gasp for air? Did you feel tightness in your throat and chest, a knot in your stomach, or maybe an ache in your back? Were your hands cool and sweaty? Did you just feel as if you couldn't wait to go to the bathroom?

If you felt some of those familiar signs of tension, you were having a sympathetic nervous system-activated "fight-or-flight" response. Of course, you had no need to fight or flee, but your body didn't know the difference between real physical danger and your more emotional reasons for uneasiness. Undoubtedly the fight-or-flight reflex once had great survival value for our cave dwelling ancestors whose primary threats were physical. Our legacy from that prehistoric period may be a supersensitive autonomic nervous system (ANS), ready to rev up the body with massive amounts of adrenaline at the slightest sign of threat. Today, for most of us, threats to our well-being aren't physical. Fighting or fleeing doesn't help much with coping with an overly tight daily schedule, oppressive job requirements, or an unhappy marriage.

Triggering the Response

Any perception of physical or emotional danger will trigger the fight-or-flight response, which is really a complex neuroendocrine set of responses that was first described by Hans Selye (1956). In response to the danger cue, the autonomic nervous system works closely with the endocrine system to supply oxygen and glucose to the blood. Muscles tighten in preparation to fight or flee. Blood vessels in the skin tighten (vasoconstrict), leaving the skin cooler. This is most evident in the hands and feet, causing them to feel cool and damp (sweaty) at the same time. Adrenalin (epinephrine) and steroid hormones are released, digestion shuts down, and respiration and heart rate speed up. These activation responses can continue to the point of total exhaustion.

Managing the Response

The fight-or-flight response is truly an amazingly effective and efficient system for preparing the body for both instant and sustained action. It isn't harmful to the body if the perceived dangers are only occasional and, once the danger is past, there is adequate time and capacity to recover.

The response, or parts of the response, can be controlled by drugs that reduce the reactivity of the central and autonomic nervous system. Although drugs may be medically necessary in some cases, it's certainly preferable to manage these stress reactions with your body's own built-in homeostatic control systems. Your response to perceived stressors can be modified by learning cognitive and physiological self-regulation exercises, thereby diminishing the effects of the fight-or-flight response. Vigorous exercise is also a good way to work off excess tension.

The Link to Headaches

The fight-or-flight response may be linked to headaches in several different ways. Headaches may be a direct result of the muscular, vascular, or neuroendocrine components of the response; the link may also be an indirect one. Repeated triggering of the response may lead to cumulative physical changes over several days that can finally lead to a headache, or lower the threshold for other headache triggers. Finally, the headache pain itself is a stressful experience that can further stimulate the body's stress response.

The Structure of Self-Regulation

Self-regulating techniques will help you to achieve a state of mental and physical calmness and to then use that calmed state to reduce the pain sensation itself. The goal is to develop a skill that can be both an "anti-fight-or-flight response" and an "anti-pain response." Self-regulation techniques are taught in various ways. However, *you will have more confidence in picking the techniques that work best for you when you understand the common features that are at the root of all self-regulation strategies, regardless of the name of the discipline.*

The basic strategies for accomplishing self-regulation are analogous to four building blocks placed on a concrete foundation. In figure 4.1, the foundation consists of *focused attention*. The key structural building blocks are as follows:

- slow-deep diaphragmatic breathing

- muscle relaxation

- hand warming

The capstone block is

- mental imagery

Focused Attention: The Foundation of Self-Regulation

The two key principles of focused attention are as follows:

1. The conscious mind can focus only on one primary event at a time.

2. The physiological functions of the body follow the primary focus of the brain.

Essentially, this means that if you can think relaxing thoughts and imagine calming, nonpainful sensations, your body will begin to follow your mind. It's a simple yet profound principle for pain control, healing, and health maintenance.

What Is "Focused Attention"?

A cognitive skill, such as focused attention, is not taught like baking a cake or changing a tire are taught. You can't learn how by watching someone else do

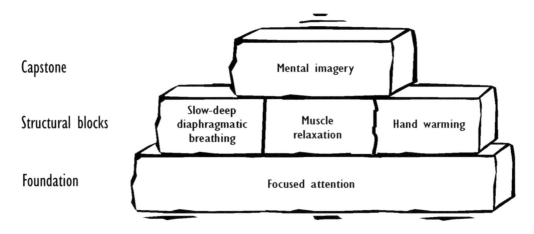

Capstone   Mental imagery

Structural blocks   Slow-deep diaphragmatic breathing   Muscle relaxation   Hand warming

Foundation   Focused attention

Figure 4.1:   **The Building Blocks of Self-Regulation**

it. Instead, to understand, you must experience it yourself. Fortunately, most of you already know how to use focused attention, even if you haven't given it much thought.

Think of your moment-by-moment thoughts, feelings, and sensations (i.e, stream of consciousness experience) as being like a TV screen or video monitor. The foreground of your screen is whatever happens to have your attention at the moment—e.g., a book, a TV show, or eating your dinner. Of course, there's always some background material on your screen, otherwise you couldn't drive while listening to the radio or converse while walking. Nevertheless, one sensation or thought will always predominate. It's virtually impossible to attend actively to more than one thing at a time—which is why cellular phones are dangerous devices in cars.

Sometimes it seems as if we are thinking about too many things at the same time. At such times, however, our attention is still *processing* only one thing at a time, but it's rapidly jumping from one idea or sensation to another. What we experience as poor attention is similar to having the foreground and background of our internal screen constantly flip-flopping. Some people seem to have been born with a very limited power of focused attention. This is the case with people who have attention deficit disorder.

When you experience poor attentional focusing, it's similar to when your car radio picks up several stations at once. At the other extreme of attention focusing is the person with the so-called one-track mind—someone who is so absorbed in a single idea that he or she has difficulty contemplating alternatives. Their internal radio never wants to scan or change stations.

Headaches and Focused Attention

The most familiar attentional problem that most of us have experienced is a preoccupation with some pressing concern. A particular worry or distressing preoccupation can seem to have a life of its own. Another familiar attentional difficulty felt by most at some time or other is the sense that our thoughts are jumping from idea to idea, never focused long enough for us to finish anything. Occasionally, the preoccupation may be positive excitement—such as anticipating an evening's events—but more often it's an intrusive worry. Such thoughts can so completely dominate our internal cognitive screen that they seem to push every possible competing thought into the background. People who wake up in the middle of the night and find themselves worrying about their job, finances, or health might recognize this problem.

A headache can take over your attention and concentration in a similar way. The headache can demand your attention even though you want to just ignore it. If it is only a dull headache, it might be compared to a small pebble in your hiking boot. You can keep on hiking despite the pebble. However, an intense, pounding headache is like trying to walk with a sharp thorn in your foot. You can't ignore it. A pounding headache so dominates your attentional screen that it wipes out all the background scenery. It becomes the loudest, clearest message, and in time, the *only* picture on your internal screen. Neurophysiologically, the headache totally dominates that part of your brain devoted to your ongoing conscious attention.

Self-regulation techniques enable you to focus your attention on other ideas and other physical functions even when you are in pain. This requires an effort to focus your attention on a station that can compete with the pain signal. Changing the station in the middle of a pounding headache isn't easy and it may seem nearly impossible. But it can be done because the competing station is playing a self-regulation message that is simple, repetitive, and easy to understand.

Think about what the following people have in common: a meditator staring at a flower; a person being "hypnotized" by a swinging pendulum; a monk or a nun counting prayer beads; or someone absorbed in a good book. Each is engaged in a cognitive process that reduces distracting thoughts by concentrating his or her attention on some external object.

Why Focused Attention Is Important

Since you can have only one thought at a time, focusing your attention on designated relaxing thoughts and images tends to block feelings and painful thoughts. Once your attention is working for you, rather than against you, you can begin to focus on imagining physical sensations that signify relaxation and health. As you become increasingly absorbed in these sensations, gradually *the physiology of your body tends to follow your mind*. That is your goal: to use your mind via focused attention to control your body.

When focused attention is used with self-regulation it's sometimes referred to as *passive concentration*. Passive concentration implies that focusing attention should be nearly effortless—you *allow* it to happen rather than *make* it happen. It's not the type of forced concentration associated with balancing a checkbook or learning a foreign language. Instead, it's a relaxed, passive generation of ideas accompanied by visual images. You don't have to act on the ideas, or solve any problems, just experience them. Passive concentration, which leads to *mental absorption*, can even have an element of pleasure, much like being absorbed by a good novel or movie.

Everyday Focused Attention

Most enjoyable daily activities are a mixture of active concentration and passive concentration/absorption. Carrying out a plan for self-regulation is no different. Monitoring the signs of tension, picking up early warning signs of a headache, and thinking about what to do, all take a certain amount of active concentration. Finding a comfortable place to rest and beginning to focus on thoughts and feelings of relaxation also requires a degree of concentrated effort. However, you should find that the active efforts of concentration will gradually move into passive concentration and then become absorption in pleasant thoughts and sensations. At that point, your cognitions will seem automatic and effortless.

Difficulties with Focused Attention

There are some circumstances that can make the basic step of narrowing your attentional focus very difficult. These include those people with

1. An attention deficit disorder with restless hyperactivity.

2. Very traumatic past experiences that remain sources of emotional conflict. Chronic tension may be a part of the effort to control these feelings and to block them from awareness.

3. Certain types of brain dysfunction due to injury, illness, or drugs that may impair ability to focus attention.

4. An inability to maintain an internal focus. Some people feel bored or anxious unless they are doing something active and their attention is focused externally. They find the self-regulation training tedious and may also demonstrate a tendency toward substance abuse to control attention.

If you have a significant problem with any of the four circumstances listed above, it could interfere with your mastering the self-regulation exercises in this book. Don't give up too soon, however, just do the best you can. If self-regulation proves to be too difficult, consider finding a therapist to help you work out a more personalized program.

If your problems with focusing attention are relatively mild, many of the exercises in this workbook can be useful for improving your cognitive capacity. Learning to be more focused on the thought or activity of the moment can be a valuable tool for helping with your headaches and may help with your ability to focus productively in other areas. People with focused-attention skills tend to get more done.

The Building Blocks of Self-Regulation

When tense, anxious, or in pain, you need to try to move the focus of your attention in the direction of a competing response. Symptoms of the fight-or-flight response can be directly reduced if you focus your attention on the four building blocks. These four strategies are essential to all efforts at stress management.

Building Block 1: Slow-Deep Diaphragmatic Breathing

Key principle: Feeling relaxed and calm requires maintaining proper blood gas balance through slow-deep diaphragmatic breathing. See figure 4.2.

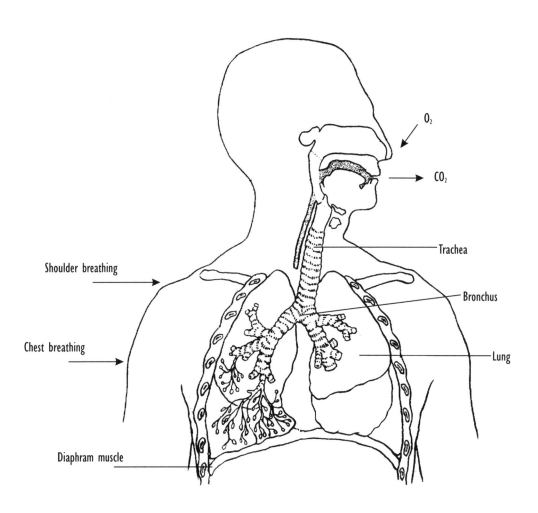

Figure 4.2:   The Mechanics of Breathing

Adapted from *The Anatomy Coloring Book* by Wynn Kapit and Lawrence M. Elson, Harper & Row, New York, 1977.

The Anatomy of Breathing

Two sets of muscles are involved in breathing. The intercostal muscles attached to the ribs, which when contracted, lift the rib cage upward and outward. The second important muscle is the diaphragm. Breathing primarily with the intercostal muscles is called high, shallow, or chest breathing, while breathing primarily with the diaphragm is called deep, diaphragmatic, or abdominal breathing. Chest breathing is an inefficient use of lung power. Although it uses more muscular energy, it fails to use the entire lung. The lower lobes of the lung may scarcely participate in the air exchange.

Take a moment to try breathing in these two different ways. First, try breathing abdominally with your diaphragm: Breathe in deeply to the count of three. Your diaphragm is tightening and pushing out your abdomen slightly. Now try breathing with your intercostal muscles, meaning rapid, shallow high chest breathing. Can you feel how inefficient this is? Anxiety often leads to rapid, shallow breathing, and this can contribute to hyperventilating.

Hyperventilation (Stress Breathing)

Both over- and underbreathing can cause blood gas (oxygen and carbon dioxide) imbalances and, ultimately, unpleasant physical symptoms. Underbreathing is more typically associated with disease states and overbreathing with stress, anxiety, and pain. Hyperventilation is the label given to overbreathing. This leads to too much carbon dioxide loss from the body (called *hypocapnia*), resulting in increased alkalinity (pH levels in the blood). Oxygen and carbon dioxide must maintain just the right balance in the blood to sustain the proper pH balance in the body. When there is an imbalance in the pH level, it can cause tension, anxiety, and fatigue. In extreme cases, the person who is hyperventilating will feel many of the symptoms of a panic attack, and may believe that he or she is on the verge of dying. These symptoms often include rapid heart rate, sweating, tingling and numbness in the limbs, tightness and pain in the chest, and eventually light-headedness and dizziness. The symptoms are often mistaken for a heart attack.

With hyperventilation, despite the overbreathing, there's a feeling of shortness of breath that leads to even more rapid, shallow chest breathing. If the breath cycle remains uncorrected, eventually, the person can pass out. Oddly enough, passing out then serves as a self-corrective measure, because with the loss of consciousness, the emotionally driven overbreathing returns to normal, and slowly allows the blood gas balance to return to normal.

Summary

Without proper blood gas levels, the organs and tissues of the body become undernourished and deteriorate. Healthy lungs and proper breathing habits are essential for good mental and physical health. Thus it's not surprising that proper breathing habits are the first rung on the ladder of self-regulation. Exercises to develop proper breathing have been part of spiritual and physical training in

Eastern cultures for centuries. In Western society, by contrast, the importance of breath control is too often ignored. Later in this chapter there are instructions for countering shallow, chest breathing by focusing your attention on slow-deep diaphragmatic breathing.

Building Block 2: Muscle Relaxation

Key principle: Feeling relaxed and calm requires a complete release of muscle tension.

Once your breathing is calm, relaxed, and diaphragmatic, it will be time to shift your attention to muscle relaxation—the next building block. Just as you can't relax while hyperventilating, you can't relax while your muscles are very tense.

Muscle Tension and Pain

The purpose of all striated muscle tissue is, by means of contraction (shortening or tensing of muscle fibers), to exert a force on the bones either for movement or to maintain upright posture. A healthy muscle is strong and flexible, capable of contracting when we want to move or maintain posture. Otherwise it should be relaxed.

The health of all muscle tissue requires a release of tension (i.e., lengthening or relaxation). A chronically tense muscle eventually will become unhealthy. If chronically tensed, the fibers of the muscle will become shorter and weaker and impair blood circulation thus allowing harmful waste products to build up in the muscle. Such a muscle may feel sore and painful, weak, or may go into spasm with even minor use.

A tense muscle is a shortened muscle. That is why muscle stretching is such a critical part of our muscle exercise routine—the muscle cannot relax if it cannot be properly lengthened.

A fundamental principle of good health is that energy expenditure should be appropriate to the demands of the situation. Your body's systems should be highly activated when you need or wish to be active, and relatively quiescent at times of relaxation and sleep. Muscles, like most other body systems, are designed to use energy and then seek rest. Muscle action is healthy for your muscles and for all other systems of your body. Problems develop when the exercise ends, but the muscle remains partially activated. In many instances when the muscle tension is not generated by actual physical demands, but rather by emotional strain, you may not even be aware the muscle is still tensed, but only of the discomfort you're feeling. A headache may be one sign of such muscle tension.

Research with people who have chronic muscular pain has demonstrated that chronically contracted muscles can become alarmingly inefficient. For example, if a healthy, pain-free individual is asked to make a tight fist while the EMG (electromyograph) muscle tension is electronically recorded from the surface of the arm, the EMG signal will be immediate and strong. But often the same signal will be sluggish and weak from a patient with pain in the muscles of the hand or arm.

Problems associated with chronic muscle tension are particularly prevalent with the antigravity muscles of the neck, back, and shoulders. These muscles can play a very important role in the origins of many headaches. When we're awake and upright, these muscles must always be activated to a certain degree. Chronic tension actually can change the structure of muscles. Chronic tension in the antigravity muscles of the upper back, neck, and head can change your posture to a degree that puts you at risk for developing chronic musculoskeletal pain and headaches (see chapter 6).

Autonomic Activation

Widespread chronic muscle tension will stimulate the autonomic nervous system (ANS) and increase neurohormonal activity. Because the chronically contracted muscles aren't sufficiently at rest, the physiological systems of the body remain activated when they should be resting. Directly and indirectly, such muscle tension effects are constant biological stressors to the body and lead to both fatigue and tension.

Naturally, a tense muscle uses more energy than a relaxed one. It's the constant demand to send more blood to tense, fatigued muscles that leaves the ANS stimulated, instead of allowing it to rest.

Muscle tension that activates the ANS connects muscle relaxation closely with the next building block, which is hand warming. Activated muscles stimulate the ANS to shunt more blood to muscles, leaving less blood available for the skin surface, and thus cooling the skin. It is one reason why our hands and feet can be so cold when we feel nervous.

Muscle Tension and Headaches

Chronic muscle tension can be involved in headaches both directly and indirectly. As you learn to regulate the muscle tension throughout your body, neck, and head, you will gain some control over your headache pain. Pain in the muscles themselves may be the source of the headache—muscles of the face, neck, and scalp may become sore and also may irritate underlying nerves and blood vessels, thus contributing to pain. Activating these same muscles may have the indirect effect of disrupting the neurochemical regulating system in the hypothalamus, which leads to some of the neurological and vascular changes that are part of the headache syndrome.

Summary

Anyone with generalized muscular tension certainly has reason to feel uncomfortable and tired. That person's body is never truly at rest and eventually becomes chronically fatigued. Increasing your awareness of the presence of tension, and becoming sensitive to the difference between tension and relaxation, is an important part of learning self-regulation.

Building Block 3: Hand and Foot Warming (Increasing Blood Flow to the Skin Surface)

Key principle: As ANS activation decreases with relaxation, a corresponding increase of blood flow to the surface of the skin increases the skin's temperature, most noticeably in the hands and feet.

The Physiology of Skin Temperature

Body heat is produced by your metabolism. Muscles produce the most heat—if you feel cold, you can warm yourself by exercising. The vascular (blood vessel) system in your body acts like a radiator. As your muscles warm up, your skin warms also. The blood absorbs heat from muscles and moves it to the skin where it can be cooled. Sweating speeds along the process of heat loss. Both tension and relaxation play a role in how blood moves throughout the body, and therefore also in the regulation of temperature.

Skin Temperature Regulation

Due to the high level of blood vessels and the density of nerve endings in the palms of the hands and fingers, it's much easier to feel temperature changes in the hands than anywhere else in the body. This is why in self-regulation training we use the term "hand warming" instead of skin temperature.

As a result of breath and muscle regulation, typically, the hands will automatically begin to warm. Hand warming can be further enhanced by *focusing attention* on feelings of warmth in the hands. This follows from the second important consequence of focused attention, namely, the body tends to follow the mind. Finally, the special contribution of hand temperature lies in its value as a gauge of ANS activation. Noticing increased warmth in your hands immediately informs you that you're successfully turning off the fight-or-flight response.

Hand Temperature and Headaches

While the effects of stress on hand temperature are nearly universal, for some people the effects are dramatic. Hand temperatures may drop several degrees from the mid-90s Fahrenheit into the high 80s, in some cases even into the 70s. Such strong reactions are more common in women than in men, suggesting a link with circulating hormones. It is noteworthy that migraine headaches also involve rapid changes in the diameter of blood vessels in the scalp and brain. It's believed that people who frequently report cold hands also tend to have more migraine headaches. Certainly, learning to warm your hands in response to stress may be a useful tool to reduce the biochemical chain of events that can lead to a blood vessel headache.

Summary

If your hands become warmer during your relaxation exercises, you know you've successfully reduced the neurohormonal activation of the fight-or-flight response. Because the body tends to follow the mind, focusing on feelings of warmth flowing into your hands can reinforce the effects of breathing and muscle relaxation.

Building Block 4: Mental Imagery

Key principles: Mental imagery is a strategy to maintain and strengthen the effects of the first three building blocks. It is a means for moving beyond mere relaxation and toward pain control.

Mental imagery comes from the imagination. In self-regulation it's not random imagining, but a conscious effort to focus on certain sensory images and physical sensations that we know can affect physiological processes in the body. Remember, the body follows the mind.

Using Imagery to Reinforce Self-Regulation

With Slow-Deep Diaphragmatic Breathing. Try to imagine seeing pure air going deep into your lungs, filling your body with life-giving oxygen. With each exhalation, imagine tension leaving your body. That tension may take a visual form, such as smoke or a cloud that drifts away. With such images, each breath cycle leaves the body feeling slightly more relaxed and calmer.

With Muscle Relaxation. Imagine your muscles as tight rubber bands, which are gradually released. You can scan your body section by section, imagining muscles in each region becoming soft and pliable like jelly, Jell-O, or sponge rubber. Or, visualize your entire body as a stiff mannequin gradually turning into a limp rag doll.

With Hand Warming. The options here are nearly endless. You might imagine your hands bathed in warm water, or lying flat against a hot rock under the hot sun. Or just imagine the sensation of warmth creeping down your arms into your hands.

Obviously no single image is the only correct one. Use whatever works best for you. Be creative. Use whatever helps to maintain that all-important focusing of your brain screen on relaxation rather than on the distracting static of troubling ideas and sensations.

Mental Imagery: Involving All Your Senses

Focusing attention via mental imaging can involve as many of your senses as you wish. For example, if imagining your hands in warm water, make the scene as simple or elaborate as you like. If you like beaches, the warm water might be the sea or a lake. Take a few moments to fill in the details. See the colors, textures, and form of water, sand, and grass. Don't forget to add sounds and smells. In addition to seeing the sun and warm water, try to feel it. Let the water be a perfect temperature. Feel the warmth soaking into your hands. By using several senses, each one reinforces the others.

Summary

Images can represent reality, modified reality, or be totally fanciful. Don't hesitate to make your images better than reality—after all this is a fantasy. Your imagined beach can be perfect, where the weather is always beautiful, the surroundings always clean, never overcrowded, and always hassle-free. Mental imaging for relaxation, better sleep, pain control, and general health can really express your individual creativity. Some people prefer their images to be realistic, e.g., relaxing in a lawn chair as opposed to floating on a cloud. Others prefer very fanciful images, e.g., tension relief as a fog that diminishes and fades away as opposed to seeing your tight muscles loosening and letting go.

Structuring the Building Blocks

Most pain and stress management techniques involve a combination of the four basic building blocks. Most forms of meditation are almost pure applications of breath control and mental imagery. Proper breathing, muscle relaxation, and hand temperature are all highly interconnected. Hyperventilation, brought on by anxiety, stimulates the ANS, which in turn tends to increase muscle tension and make the hands colder by drawing blood away from the skin. Conversely, to relax and replenish the muscles and calm the autonomic nervous system, you need to have an adequate oxygen and carbon dioxide balance leading to a proper pH balance. Anything short of this goal leads to increase risk of discomfort, poorer health, and headaches.

The (BMW)I Formula: Self-Regulation Steps to Remember

It always helps memory to condense ideas into a kind of shorthand. As you begin working with self-regulating techniques, you may find it convenient to remember that focused attention is placed on:

B reath = Slow-deep breathing

M uscle = Muscle relaxation

W arm = Warming hands (skin)

I magery = Imagery (mental)

Once you are skilled at self-monitoring and self-regulating, a quick scan of your breathing, muscle tension, and hand temperature (warmth) becomes as easy as checking the temperature, pressure, and fuel gauges of your car. The entire process can be summarized as SCAN, FOCUS, and (BMW)I. The I is set apart from the parenthesis to indicate it applies equally to all three building blocks.

Key Word Summary for Section I

To ensure that you have thoroughly mastered the material in this section, write the definition of each term below in your own words. Future chapters will build on your understanding of these terms.

Focused attention: _____
_____
_____

Passive concentration: _____
_____
_____

Mental absorption: _____
_____
_____

Fight-or-flight response: _____
_____
_____

Autonomic nervous system (ANS): _____
_____
_____
_____

Hyperventilation: _____
_____
_____

pH level: _____
_____
_____

Mental imagery: _____
_____
_____

(BMW)I formula: _____
_____
_____

Section II: Using the Building Blocks

Self-Monitoring: Using a Stress/Tension Body Scan

A major part of managing headaches is not to let them sneak up on you. Be alert to early warning signs, or to subtle indications of tension in your neck or back, around your eyes and mouth, or in your throat and chest. Watch for other fight-or-flight physical indicators. Be on the lookout for whatever happens to be your own unique signature of stress—tightness in your throat or chest, sweating, cold hands, or a feeling of jitteriness, or loss of concentration—anything that is a cue that it is time to use your (BMW)I relaxation skills.

Some people aren't very good at stress monitoring because they have become so accustomed to chronic physical and mental stress they simply don't recognize the stress symptoms. If this sounds familiar, it can be helpful to conduct a brief stress inventory at least once an hour. For the first few days, set your watch to beep on the hour to remind you to do a quick body scan for signs of stress.

Keeping written records can also be a helpful reminder. Simple logs, using the type of ten-point rating scale described in chapter 3 for rating headache pain, work well for most people. You may want to make a list of three or four most common stress indicators and rate them three or four times a day such as shown in the sample stress log provided in chapter 3.

Note that just as there are headache triggers, so too there are *relaxation triggers*. A cue word, phrase, or image can become the tool to make a quick shift from an activity to a state of focused attention.

How to Do the Exercises

Whenever you see the ✱ symbol, specific instructions will follow. All scripts are set in italics. With practice you can try to work with the script from memory. When you're getting started, it may be easier to have someone read the script to you. Or you could read it into a tape recorder and play the tape to guide your self-regulation efforts. The advantage of using a tape early in your practice is that it helps you to maintain focused attention.

✱ Script: Switching Focus

Imagine you are standing on the top of a hill where you see a doorway or a gate in a stone or brick wall. You approach the gate and see printed on it the word "RELAX." This is the gate through which you can enter your self-regulation world.

> 1. *As you imagine yourself moving through the gate, say (or think) to yourself the cue word on the gate. Or think of such phrases as, "This is my moment for comfort and peace, it is my time to let go."*

2. *On the other side of the gate, you find yourself in a small patio or garden overlooking a beautiful landscape. You find a comfortable reclining chair from which you can view the landscape beyond. It's a view you immediately associate with feeling calm, serene, and secure. The scene can be as elaborate or simple as you wish. It might be a pasture or a meadow that slopes down to a peaceful stream. It could be a beach, lake, or ocean. It could have palm trees rustling in a gentle breeze, or it could be your own backyard. In fact, it doesn't even have to be an outdoor scene at all. It could be a special room you associate with feeling mentally calm and totally relaxed.*

3. *Once you are there, take a seat, and settle down. It is time to shift your focus to slow-deep breathing.*

Remember, there's no "correct" mental imagery. The suggestions above are just that— suggestions. The process of the attentional focusing is what is critical, not the specific content of the images.

Cue-controlled Relaxation

With cueing, you are practicing what learning theorists call *stimulus-response conditioning*. If you feel relaxed following certain words, thoughts, or images, over time that cue can alone trigger the relaxation response. In the language of learning theory, the cue becomes a *classically conditioned stimulus*, which elicits the *conditioned response* of relaxation and pain relief. This principle of cue association is used by advertisers all the time to get us to behave in ways that are good for their businesses. Here is a chance to use this principle to your own advantage.

A cue has the advantage of being quick and adaptable to any setting—in the office, at the dinner table, even while driving. The amount of detail you put into the imaginary scene depends on time and circumstance. If you have a lot of time, you can increase your degree of absorption into the imaginary scene by adding further detail. Remember, you can add details to your script from your other senses. When constructing your script, notice all the colors, smells, and textures. Pay special attention to the feelings of temperature, sun, and breeze on your skin.

Don't strain for all these details. Allow them to just float into your mind. The more you get into the scene, the more your senses are involved, the easier it will become. The more relaxed and focused your attention becomes, the easier it will be to move from the cognitive to the more physical components of self-regulation.

Focusing on the (BMW)I Building Blocks

Once you have used the gate image (or an equivalent) to complete your shift of focus, you're ready to follow the four-pronged (BMW)I self-regulation exercise.

Block I: Slow-Deep Diaphragmatic Breathing

Establishing a pattern of comfortable slow-deep breathing is the single most critical element of self-regulation. That is why "B" is listed first in the (BMW)I formula. It's the fastest and most direct route available for directly influencing the fundamental biochemistry of your body, and thus is the most powerful tool you have to counter the effects of stress. Sit in a comfortable chair in the most comfortable position you can assume and even if you have trouble focusing your attention go ahead and give slow-deep breathing your best shot.

✱ Script: Simple Quick Breath Control

You already know how important diaphragmatic breathing is to maintaining proper blood gas balance. When stressed, you may tend towards rapid, shallow overbreathing. This can increase your feelings of stress and make a headache even worse.

1. *Place one hand on your stomach and the other hand on your chest. Think the words "slow-deep-smooth."*

2. *Inhale slowly through your nostrils for three full seconds. Then exhale for another three seconds. (Note that you can count seconds by saying "one-one thousand, two-one thousand, three-one thousand" to yourself to complete a full three seconds.) The hand on your abdomen should move more than the hand on your chest—remember, you're breathing primarily using your diaphragm.*

3. *Count out another full two seconds before you start your next breath. Keep it as smooth as possible. Feel the tension leave your body as you exhale.*

4. *Let your breathing become automatic. The counting is only to help you create the rhythm. Occasionally, return to your breathing cue thoughts: slow-deep-smooth.*

The breath cycle should look like the illustration in figure 4.3. You may find it helpful to remember this picture while you focus on your breathing. Your cue words are: **slow-deep-smooth**.

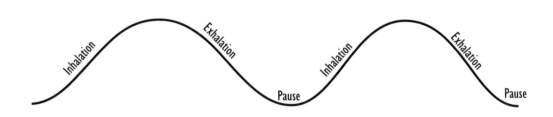

Figure 4.3:   **The Breathing Cycle**

Supplementary Breath Control Scripts

A few simple instructions, such as those expressed in the preceding script, are usually all it takes to establish a comfortable, proper breathing pattern, and I do not want to overwhelm you with information when simple instructions will do. However, you should be aware that there is a great deal of additional written information available on this topic. Below are three examples of other deep-breathing tips adapted from *The Relaxation & Stress Reduction Workbook* and *The Chronic Pain Control Workbook*.

✳ <u>Script:</u> Increasing Breathing Awareness

1. *Lie down on a rug or blanket on the floor with your legs uncrossed and slightly apart. See figure 4.4. Allow your arms to relax comfortably at your sides. Close your eyes.*

2. *Focus your attention on your breathing and place one hand on the part of your body that seems to rise and fall the most as you inhale and exhale. Note that if this spot is in your chest, you are not making good use of the lower part of your lungs. People who are nervous or in pain tend to breathe many short, shallow breaths in their upper chest.*

3. *Place both of your hands gently on your abdomen and follow your breathing. Notice how your abdomen rises with each inhalation and falls with each exhalation.*

4. *Allow yourself to breathe through your nose. Clear your nasal passages before doing breathing exercises.*

5. *Check if your chest is moving in harmony with your abdomen, or if it is rigid.*

6. *As you breathe comfortably, scan your body for tension, especially in your throat, chest, and abdomen.*

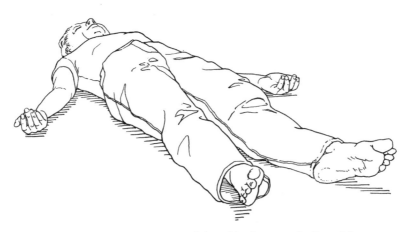

Figure 4.4:   **A Good Position for Practicing Diaphragmatic Breathing**

✱ <u>Script</u>: Slow-Deep Abdominal Breathing—Sitting or Standing

Proper, healthy breathing can be practiced anywhere—in the office, riding a bus, prior to bedtime, or after you have gone to bed—while sitting, standing, or lying down. To become comfortable with the technique, it's recommended that you first practice while lying on your back. Once slow-deep abdominal breathing becomes automatic for you, it will take only seconds to use it anywhere and anytime to help relieve your tension and pain.

1. *Focus your attention on a body scan for signs of tension, pain, and rapid, shallow breathing.*

2. *Sit or stand in as comfortable a position as possible.*

3. *Inhale slowly through your nostrils. Feel the breath move through your chest down to your stomach.*

4. *Hold for a second and then reverse the process, allowing the breath to pass back out through your chest and nostrils. As you exhale, feel your muscles let go of tension. Allow your jaw to unclench and your neck to relax as you exhale.*

✱ <u>Script</u>: Slow-Deep Abdominal Breathing—on Your Stomach

This is a useful exercise especially if you have difficulty feeling the movement of your diaphragm while breathing in a sitting or lying down position.

1. *Lie on your stomach, placing your legs a comfortable distance apart with your toes pointed outward. Fold your arms in front of your body, resting your hands on your biceps. Position your arms so that your chest doesn't touch the floor.*

2. *As you inhale, feel your abdomen pressing against the floor. As you slowly exhale, feel your abdominal muscles relaxing. It is easy to feel the diaphragmatic motion in this position.*

Block 2: Muscle Relaxation

It's time to turn your attention to the next critical building block of self-regulation—muscle relaxation. This is the "M" in the (BMW)I formula.

✱ <u>Script</u>: Simple-Quick Muscle Relaxation

As you continue to breathe slowly and deeply, let your attention move to your muscles.

1. *Begin by making mental contact with the muscles of your jaw and neck because these areas of the body become tense easily. Does your jaw feel tight?*

Let all the tension out of the jaw. Your mouth can be closed, but your teeth shouldn't be touching. Let that feeling of relaxation spread to where the jaw muscles fan out above your ears. (See figure 4.5.) With each exhalation, feel more and more tension leave your muscles, almost as if you were slowly letting the air out of a balloon. With each inhalation replace the tension with more and more relaxation.

2. *Add imagery. Imagine that you have Jell-O throughout your body instead of muscles.*

3. *Let this wonderful, pleasant feeling of relaxation flow down from your neck, into your shoulders, right on through your shoulder joints into your upper arms, all the way to your elbows, and then all the way down your forearms into your hands and fingers. Maybe you'll find that the relaxation moves through your body rapidly, or maybe it just creeps along slowly, just an inch or two with each breath. Give into the pleasant feeling of relaxed heaviness as more and more individual muscles release their tension and ease into total, calm relaxation. It's a relaxed heaviness you feel, especially in your arms, not a fatigued heaviness, because your muscles are becoming so limp that it feels as if it would take great effort to move them.*

4. *Let the flow of relaxation continue through your chest into your abdomen, and into the muscles of your pelvis and buttocks, into your thighs and finally all the way down your legs, through your knee joints and ankles and into your feet. Continue to make mental contact with your arms and legs and repeat to yourself, "Relaxed heaviness is flowing into my arms, relaxed heaviness is flowing into my legs, relaxed heaviness is flowing into my arms and legs."*

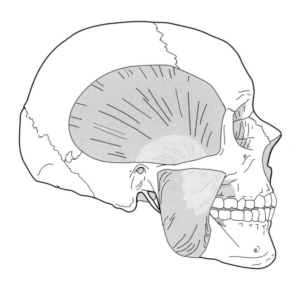

Figure 4.5:   The Muscles of Mastication

As you become deeply relaxed, you might notice that one or more of your limbs feel almost disconnected from your body. It may even feel as if your body parts are floating off into space. If you have such an experience, don't worry. This can happen when muscles are so profoundly relaxed that they send very few neural signals to the brain. It's like parts of your body are sleeping and your brain has lost track of where they are.

More Muscle Relaxation Scripts

The simple-quick relaxation exercise presented above is considered a *passive* muscle relaxation technique. If you found it easy to become deeply relaxed, you are ready to move on to hand warming. But if you feel as if you need more work on muscle relaxation, turn to the appendix for more scripts for both active and passive muscle relaxation strategies. Then, return to hand warming below when you feel ready.

Block 3: Hand Warming (Increasing Blood Flow to the Skin)

We turn now to the "W" in the (BMW)I in the self-regulation formula. This building block often becomes automatic as a result of your breath and muscle regulation. So why include it at all? The answer is that hand temperature is very useful to gauge the tension in your muscles. If your hand temperature is increasing, you know that you are accomplishing your goal of achieving physiologic relaxation effects from your cognitive focusing. Thus W, for warmth, is included as the third critical element in the building block formula.

If you have cold hands and feet from pain or nervous tension, it will be rewarding to feel them change. As a self-regulator, it's like your perfect home run.

In addition, for medical conditions where peripheral blood flow is impaired, enhancing blood flow is useful to nourish the tissue of the hands and feet. One of the most dramatic and rewarding events of my twenty-five years in teaching self-regulation occurred when a man with highly ulcerous feet due to poor circulation, who was facing possible amputation for gangrene, was able to restore his feet to health with foot warming training.

✳ Script: Simple Quick Hand Warming

Now that your breathing is calm and relaxed and all the tension has drained from your muscles, move your attention to your hands for a few moments. How do they feel? Are they relaxed, very limp, and fully supported by the arms of the chair? Do they feel warm and have they been getting warmer as you become more and more relaxed? As your muscles become more relaxed, they require less blood. Therefore, more blood can go to the surface of the skin. This makes the skin warmer. You can best feel this increased warmth from the blood coming to the skin in your hands. The hands are very sensitive because they have so many sensory nerve endings compared to many other parts of the skin. If more blood is flowing to your hands, you may begin to feel a slight tingling sensation in your palms and fingers. Also, you might feel a very slight swelling in your fingers and perhaps a very faint pulse. Sometimes you can help the warming process along by imagining warmth flowing into your hands. Or imagine your hands are immersed in warm water or basking in direct sunlight. Don't be too concerned about what temperature they actually are, but focus instead on imagining or remembering what warmth feels like. If you can imagine the feeling, your body tends to follow your mind.

1. *Direct your attention to your hands. Are they relaxed and warm? Have they been getting warmer?*

2. *Imagine what warmth feels like. Even if your hands seem cold, try to focus on how warmth would feel.*

3. *Imagine your hands in warm water or make up another warm scene.*

Supplementary Hand Warming Script

Now suggestions of warmth are interspersed with suggestions of heaviness. Note that the exercises always begin with the phrase, "My right arm is heavy."

* Script: Autogenic Hand and Foot Warming

My right arm is heavy.
My arms and legs are heavy.
My right arm is warm.
My left arm is warm.
Both of my arms are warm.

* *My right arm is heavy.*
My arms and legs are heavy.
My right arm is warm.
My left arm is warm.
My right leg is warm.
Both of my legs are warm.
My arms and legs are warm.

* *My right arm is heavy.*
My arms and legs are heavy.
Both of my arms are warm.
Both of my legs are warm.
My arms and legs are warm.
My arms and legs are heavy and warm.

* *My right arm is heavy.*
My arms and legs are heavy.
My arms and legs are warm.
My arms and legs are heavy and warm.

Notes on Hand Warming

If you encounter difficulty achieving hand warming, it is wise to step back and return to muscle relaxation. Try not to worry about it. Any frustration, self-criticism, or competing thoughts or emotions that stir up the sympathetic nervous system activity will block the warming response. It's truly one of those physiological responses for which you can *set the stage* and *allow* it to happen, but you can't actually *make* it happen. As soon as you get frustrated and try too hard, the temperature will move in the opposite direction.

Hands get warmer, then colder. If you are doing (BMW)I self-regulation in a room with a normal temperature, you may be perplexed when your hand temperature steadily rises for eight or ten minutes, but thereafter begins to decline even though you continue to feel very relaxed. What you're observing is the temperature regulation reflex in action. Keep in mind that the vasoconstriction of the small blood vessels near the skin surface is not only a product of stress, but is also an internal body temperature regulation reflex.

Warmer skin temperatures for eight or ten minutes followed by a cooling temperature is a commonplace occurrence because relaxed muscles produce little body heat. If completely relaxed, it may take only a few minutes, even at normal room temperature, to begin to become slightly chilled. At that point, vasoconstriction occurs at the skin in an effort to keep internal body temperature at a constant 98.6°F. That's why you need a sheet or blanket over you while sleeping even in a moderately warm room. Because this temperature preservation reflex overrides the relaxation effect, only the first few minutes of the session really reflect the relaxation effect. One option is to wear an extra sweater or to cover yourself with a blanket while practicing self-regulation.

Block 4: Mental Imagery

Now you will move your attention to the "I" outside the parentheses, the final component of the (BMW)I formula. You have already been using imagery with the BMW focusing, but now you can go farther with it to strengthen the breath, muscle, and warming components of self-regulation.

Using Imagery to Support BMW Physiological Self-Regulation

❊ Script: With Slow-Deep Breathing

With each exhalation continue to feel the tension leave your body. You may find it helpful to actually imagine seeing the clean air going deep into your lungs and spreading from your lungs throughout your body with each inhalation. Then, imagine a kind of foggy exhaust filled with tension fumes leaving your body with each exhalation. As the tension fumes leave your body, imagine that the fog gradually thins, until eventually the exhaled air is nearly as clear as the incoming air.

✱ <u>Script</u>: With Muscle Relaxation

Imagine the muscles in your neck tightly knotted up like a wash cloth that you are trying to wring out. With each exhalation, imagine that wash cloth loosens up a little bit more until finally it's returned to its normal flat, open state—just as your muscles become longer and flatter as they become increasingly more comfortable. Or, imagine your entire body as a stiff mannequin gradually turning into a limp rag doll.

✱ <u>Script</u>: With Hand Warming

Imagine your hands immersed in warm water, resting in the sunlight, or on a heating pad. Or just imagine warmth creeping down your arms into your hands. If you're comfortable with internal body images, imagine blood vessels near your skin opening and filling with rich, red blood. Or imagine that your hands and feet are changing from a cold, bluish-gray color to a healthy, warm, pinkish color.

Application to Headaches

In the next chapter we will consider further applications of mental imagery to headaches. With mental imagery, many people can go beyond relaxation to experience partial or, in rare instances, complete analgesia. This is done primarily by focusing on sensations that directly compete with the pain. It is important to understand that such a high degree of mind control over physical sensation becomes possible when you understand and can fully use all of the building blocks contained within the (BMW)I formula.

The (BMW)I Self-Regulation Formula

The (BMW)I formula that simply summarizes the building blocks of self-regulation can be your cue for easily remembering the key elements of self-regulation. It can take some of the mystery out of what otherwise may seem to be exotic exercises. Ideally, in time, you will find you can do the basic steps automatically and they will require little effort.

Fitting the Parts into the Whole

Review how the building blocks fit together into the whole picture of mind-body relaxation. Your focus on breathing can be combined with an awareness of body position, a letting go of muscle tension, and a feeling of warmth flowing into your hands. In time, you may feel these things happening automatically. At first it might feel like learning to drive a stick shift, where you first focus on parts of the movement, but in time the actions become automatic, based on a feel for the whole rather than a focus on the separate components.

"How much time is it going to take to do the (BMW)I training?" is a familiar question. Regrettably, "I just don't have the time" is the most common excuse expressed for not practicing self-regulation exercises, just as it is for physical exercise.

The key to managing the time requirements is to avoid becoming too rigid about what you must do—just as it is better to spend only ten or fifteen minutes a day in physical exercise than not do any at all. If you cannot try at all because you cannot attain a higher ideal, you are too idealistic. Ultimately, (BMW)I is not just a matter of how much you formally practice, but also a matter of very practical daily activities such as how you ride the bus, sit at your desk, and eat your dinner.

When you're just getting started, two practice sessions a day of approximately twenty to thirty minutes each is ideal. But you can shorten the sessions to as little as five minutes a day, if that is all the time you have. Although some therapists will recommend much more time than this, remember that anything is better than nothing. It may be helpful to think of time and depth of practice in terms of minimum and maximum applications.

Time and Depth of Practice

Each episode of self-regulation practice can be rated on the *time* spent and the *depth* of relaxation achieved. Depending on your time and circumstances, each effort will fall somewhere on the minimum vs. maximum continuum.

	Minimum	vs.	Maximum
Time:	brief	vs.	lengthy
Depth:	limited	vs.	profound

Maximum Application of Self-Regulation

For a maximum session, *lengthy* might be twenty to thirty minutes. *Profound* would be a state of full-body relaxation in a comfortable reclining chair or bed that completely supports the body. The goal is to achieve a feeling of peacefulness where it truly feels as if the body is asleep even though the mind can still observe. This is the Holy Grail of self-regulated relaxation.

Minimum Application of Self-Regulation

Brief and *limited* self-regulation is what you do while driving, at your desk, or when talking on the telephone. If reduced muscle tension and lowered autonomic/neuroendocrine activation are to become part of your daily life, using these minimum applications is critical. Do a quick scan of your breathing, muscles, and hands. Smooth out your breathing, let go of excessive tension in your jaw and neck, imagine warmth flowing into your hands while you continue to do whatever you are doing. While driving, for example, you need to maintain just enough muscle tension to sit up and control the steering wheel, but your entire body needn't be wrapped in muscle tension. Excessive muscle tension in your jaw, neck, and chest does not make you any safer or more alert. It just makes you feel fatigued and may cause a headache.

Midway Application of Self-Regulation

Midway between the two extremes of minimum and maximum application might be a five-minute break where you retreat to a quiet comfortable place for a quick stress scan followed by the complete (BMW)I self-regulation routine. A great deal can be accomplished in two to five minutes to adjust blood gas, muscle tension, and neurohormonal activation. Remember, the more often you practice, the quicker and easier self-regulation becomes.

Work Around Tension and Pain Blockages

As you move the focus of your attention over your body, especially during muscle relaxation, do not become bogged down by persistent tough spots. For example, while letting relaxation flow down from your head and neck into your arms, if you encounter a persistent knot of pain or tension at some point in your shoulder, just let the feeling of relaxation flow around it. Maybe you can return at a later point.

Unpleasant but Rare Side Effects

The vast majority of people find practicing self-regulation to be enjoyable. Most people experience improvement in their sense of well-being. There are, however, a few rare side effects of which you should be aware.

1. Loss of awareness of body parts. The most common of these rare problems is the loss of awareness of the body or position. With profound muscle relaxation, there is a reduction in proprioceptive feedback (the reception of stimuli) to the brain. If you close your eyes for a moment and raise your arms to a horizontal or upright vertical position, you can still sense their exact location in space. But with your arms in a supported resting position, reduction in muscle tension may cause them to feel as if they're floating or have disappeared. You have to peek to see if your arms are still there. Some people may feel as if their body is evaporating and various parts are floating away. Usually, just opening your eyes or moving slightly will take care of the problem, but a therapist should be alerted to this phenomenon and know what to do to minimize it for those who find it disturbing.

2. Parasympathetic rebound. Occasionally, an individual who is very good at self-regulation will suddenly feel quite ill. This can include nausea, vomiting, vertigo, headache, and possibly rapid onset of aches and pains. Usually, this problem can be eliminated by slowing down the process of relaxation. Keep your eyes open and sit in an upright position, even move around for ten or fifteen seconds if necessary. Let the process of relaxation settle in very gradually.

3. Autogenic abreactions. The literature frequently mentions something called *autogenic abreaction.* This appears to be a sudden onset of physical symptoms following relaxation very much like that described as parasympathetic rebound, but it also can be accompanied by a sudden release of emotions that may feel overwhelming in the moment. Quite suddenly a person may burst into tears with little clue as to why.

   This sudden release of emotions is very difficult to understand. One guess is that in some individuals, chronic muscle tension plays the role of keeping a "lid" on feelings and memories, and a rather abrupt release of the physical tension removes this emotional lid. It is likely to be only a temporary problem, but if persistent, a therapist should be consulted.

4. Need for medication adjustments. If you're taking medication for any condition related to the functioning of the ANS or endocrine systems, self-regulation may influence (usually reduce) your need for medication. This has been reported for those taking blood pressure, heart, or thyroid medications, or insulin for diabetes. Certainly we hope that it is the case for pain medications. If you're on any medications for chronic conditions, make sure to check with your doctor for any necessary adjustments.

Note to the Reader

By now you must be eager to move on and begin the direct application of self-regulation techniques to headaches. You should feel free to do so at this time, unless you are having great difficulty with the effort to allow your muscles to become fully relaxed. If that is the case, spend some time practicing with the scripts in the appendix. Because the easing of muscle tension is so important to success for both general relaxation and headache management, the extra effort will be worth your time. For those of you ready to move on to the next chapter, it may be useful to come back to this section periodically to refresh your knowledge and skill in muscle relaxation.

Key Word Summary for Section II

To ensure that you have thoroughly mastered the material in this section, write the definition of each term below in your own words. Future chapters will build on your understanding of these terms.

SCAN: _____

_____

_____

FOCUS: _____

_____

_____

(BMW)I: _____

_____

_____

MINIMUM: _____

_____

_____

MAXIMUM: _____

_____

_____

Partial relaxation: _____

_____

_____

Autogenic phrases: _____

_____

_____

Further Reading

Benson, H. and E. Stuart. 1992. *The Wellness Book: The Comprehensive Guide to Maintaining Health and Treating Stress-Related Illness*. Secaucus, NJ: Birch Lane Press.

Catalano, E. and K. Hardin. 1996. *The Chronic Pain Control Workbook*. 2d ed. Oakland, CA: New Harbinger Publications, Inc.

Davis, M., E. R. Eschelman, and M. McKay. 1995. *The Relaxation & Stress Reduction Workbook*. 4th ed. Oakland, CA: New Harbinger Publications, Inc.

Fried, R. 1987. *The Hyperventilation Syndrome: Research and Clinical Treatment*. Baltimore: The Johns Hopkins University Press.

Hafen, B. Q., K. J. Frandsen, K. J. Karren, and K. R. Hooker. 1992. *The Health Effects of Attitudes, Emotions, and Relationships*. Provo, Utah: EMS Associates.

Hollandsworth, J. J., Jr. 1986 *Physiology and Behavioral Therapy*. New York: Plenum.

Jacobson, E. 1974. *Progressive Relaxation*. Chicago: The University of Chicago Press, Midway Reprint.

Kabat-Zinn, J. 1990. *Full Catastrophe Living*. New York: Dell.

Selye, H. 1956. *The Stress of Life*. New York: McGraw-Hill.

Smith, J. C. 1989. *Relaxation Dynamics*. Champaign, IL: Research Press.

CHAPTER 5

Ending the Pain

In chapter 4 you learned the *why* and *how* of self-regulation. This chapter applies the (BMW)I self-regulation formula to your headaches. The essentials of self-regulating your headaches consist of the application of the (BMW)I relaxation response and mental imagery to

1. The *prevention* of headaches

2. The *reduction* of severity when headaches do occur

3. The improvement of *tolerance* of pain even when headache pain is severe.

Combating Headache with Self-Regulation

If you want to review the details of the SCAN, FOCUS, (BMW)I strategy for steps 1–4, turn back to chapter 4.

Step 1. SCAN. Carry out a frequent self-monitoring stress/tension scan. If you're going to break the pattern of controlling cognitive and physical tension before it turns into a headache, you must be aware of tension as it develops.

Step 2. Set the stage for relaxation. If possible, find a quiet place with a comfortable chair with adequate head and armrests. If such a place isn't available, prepare to do what you can wherever you are.

Step 3. FOCUS. Use an attention-focusing word, such as "calm," as you cross an imaginary gateway to a pleasant, secure, relaxed place.

Step 4. (BMW)I. Go through as much of your (BMW)I self-regulation formula as your circumstances allow. (Another brief sample script appears at end of this chapter.)

<u>Step 5.</u> Intensified imagery. If you're calm and physically relaxed but headache pain persists, try to go further with your mental focusing with the imagery alternatives described in this chapter.

<u>Step 6.</u> End of session. If your time is up, or you feel as relaxed as you want to be, open your eyes and slowly shift your focus to the other side of the imagined gate. Carry with you as much of the relaxed feeling and mental calmness as you can to this side of the gate. Continue to self-monitor. How long can you hold onto the feeling of relaxation, or at least part of it?

You've just completed a brief self-regulation relaxation session. That's all you'll need to do. Doing this five to fifteen minute (BMW)I routine whenever your self-scan tells you that your tension is rising can smooth out the muscular and neuroendocrine ups and downs that may lead to headaches. Because imagery is used to support both the basic relaxation effort and the headache analgesia, you should intensify your use of imagery when you need to.

More Headache Self-Regulating Techniques

If a headache has already begun before you start your self-regulation session, a minor headache may be cut short with steps 1–4 of the relaxation routine. However, if you're in the throes of a severe headache, a deeper journey into mental imagery might be required to produce some pain relief.

This involves imagining vivid sensations that directly compete with your headache.

✱ Script: Option 1—Pain-fading Imagery

Now that your breathing is calm, your muscles are relaxed, and your hands feel warm, you can do more to fade your headache into the background of your attentional screen. You may have already noticed as you focused your attention on your arms, hands, or feet that your headache may have faded slightly into the background. That's because your brain can pay really close attention to only one thing at a time. If you focus on or make contact with one part of your body, everything else tends to fade—at least a little. This doesn't come easy with a bad headache. Be curious—see what you can do.

You can go even farther with the idea of fading. Direct your attention to some part of your body that feels fine (e.g., your right foot). Think about how relaxed, comfortable, and warm it feels. For a moment take notice of some of the sensations in this foot you would usually ignore. Observe the texture of the sock against your skin. Feel how your foot fits perfectly into your shoe. Take note of the slight pressure of the shoe around your foot. Are there any pressure points from the shoe? Can you notice a feeling of warmth and a slight tingling in your toes?

Take a deep breath and as you slowly let it out, let that good feeling from your foot move up into your lower leg, into your calf, right through your knee and into your upper leg and thigh, and from your leg on into your lower abdomen. Let the good feeling keep moving right on up. With each breath, let that warm, comfortable feeling move a little higher until it has moved through your stomach, your chest, and right on into your throat, up to your jaw. Traveling upward, this calm, pleasant, relaxed sensation moves from your jaw and spreads through your entire head as if it wants to push the headache right out through the top of your head. Let that good feeling surround the headache, sweep it aside, and absorb it. Can you feel it shrink the size or lighten the weight of your headache?

✱ Script: Option 2—Counterstimulation Imagery

Imagine a cool, damp cloth resting on your head (or use an actual cool, damp cloth). Imagine this cloth has great power. It has a perfect texture. It feels silky smooth on your forehead. Its cool dampness is just the perfect temperature to relieve your discomfort. It feels so good it's almost like magic. Because you're using your imagination it can, in fact, be magic. So imagine it's a magical healing cloth and the good feeling it creates soaks right into your skin, into your scalp, and it soothes all your head muscles. Irritated blood vessels and nerves become relaxed, calmed, and cooled. With each breath the comfort sinks in a little deeper. It may seem strange that you can feel pain and pleasant, cool relief at the same time; it's almost as if the good-feeling nerves are battling the bad-feeling nerves. With each breath let the good-feeling nerves advance a little more, and push those bad-feeling nerves more and more off to the side. Let the pain fade a little bit more. Maybe you can feel the throbbing discomfort fade to more of a mild pressure, something you may not like but certainly can tolerate. With each breath let out just a little bit more pain. See how far away you can push the pain.

✱ Script: Option 3—Symbolic Representation Imagery

Try to imagine your headache as a thing you can see, for example, a colored disc, a balloon, or a dark cloud. With each exhalation of a relaxed breath, see in your mind's eye the colored disc shrinking in size and becoming lighter in color, or the balloon deflating, or the cloud rising and fading away.

✱ Script: Option 4—Distraction Imagery

Visualize a safe, secure, pleasant place you would love to be right now. What do you see there? Imagine as much detail as you can; use textures, color, and aromas. Feel yourself really become a part of that pleasant place.

✱ Script: Option 5—Autogenic Phrases

Repeat in your mind several times:
My right arm is heavy.
My right arm is warm.
My arms and legs are heavy and warm.
My whole body feels heavy, comfortable, and relaxed.
My mind is quiet.
My forehead is cool.

After your mind feels quiet and your forehead feels cool, add the additional phrase:
My pain is easing up.

Comments on Intensified Imagery

You may recognize that these headache scripts are using imagery to give the pain some competition within the sensory cortex of your brain. Pain is a loud, attention-grabbing signal to the brain, and a headache can be among the loudest and most obnoxious of signals. By shifting your attention to other sensations, you're trying to give the pain signal some competition within the sensory cortex.

Script Option 1 is a *pain-fading* technique that uses focusing on a nonpainful part of your body to try to move the headache from the dominant foreground position on your attentional screen to the background.

Script Option 2 gives your headache *counterstimulation* (or competition) by applying a relief-giving fantasy stimulus directly to the painful part of your body. It can also be done by applying actual physical counterstimulation, e.g., the cool, damp cloth on your forehead, and then by bolstering the cool cloth effect with imagery.

Script Option 3 represents the pain as a fantasy symbol of pain—as a color, cloud, or balloon—and then alters the symbol by imagination. Remember, your body tends to follow your mind, even if the mental image is only a *symbolic representation* of the pain.

Script Option 4 is a pure *distraction fantasy*, not a direct effort at an actual sensory change. Sometimes, when you are frustrated by the fact that it's just too difficult to change the headache sensation at all, it may be easier to focus on an image that is pleasant, relaxing, and calm but has nothing at all to do with your headache.

Script Option 5 uses *autogenic phrases*. These simple, repetitive phrases can be useful in focusing attention on the type of sensation you wish to feel. In this case, you are attempting to contrast your headache with pleasant feelings in other areas of your body to help ease the pain. (For more autogenic exercises, see the appendix.)

Self-Regulation and the Different Types of Headaches

Fortunately, you don't have to learn a different set of self-regulation techniques for each type of headache. Nevertheless, there are some differences in how the techniques fit with the differing patterns of headaches.

Common Features of All Headaches

All of the self-regulating strategies described in this workbook are intended to promote general cognitive and physiological relaxation. They can be useful for any type of head and neck pain. Most people find that if they can intentionally make themselves feel more relaxed; it's like turning down the "pain volume." A common report is that "the pain is still there, but it no longer controls me and sets my nerves on edge."

It's important that you think of these exercises as learning *coping skills* to improve self-management of your headaches, rather than as *treatments*. These are skills to be used whenever your pain or feelings of tension become disruptive. Having these skills can reduce the fear of pain, and allow you to attempt activities that you might have been avoiding because you were afraid a headache would result. Finally, if you can achieve a relaxed mind/body state, it becomes much easier to actually use mental imagery to ease your pain. The following types of headaches have already been described in chapter 2, but now they are related to self-regulation.

Tension Headaches

Even though muscle tightness and spasm are not the whole story behind the symptoms associated with tension headaches, there's ample reason to believe that controlling muscle tension can be useful in managing tension headaches. Thus the rationale for using self-regulating strategies to treat tension headaches is quite simple. If you can learn to prevent or reduce the tightness of the muscles of your head, neck, and upper torso, it follows that by so doing you can prevent, or at least reduce, the pain coming from these areas.

Of all stress-related symptoms, situational tension headaches are probably the most responsive to self-regulation. By quickly releasing your tension at the first sign of discomfort in your neck, jaw, or scalp, you may be able virtually to eliminate this type of headache. But you must remember to self-monitor and try to catch the tension buildup early.

Migraine Headaches

Migraine headaches are more difficult to control than tension headaches, and the rationale for using self-regulating skills to counter migraine or other vascular headaches is more complex. In fact, using relaxation as a counterheadache response may contradict the intuitive experience of many migraine sufferers. Migraine patients often report the paradoxical experience of feeling the onset of a headache during times of low stress—while sleeping, on weekends, or on vacation. If you are a task-oriented individual, who faces frequent deadlines, these paradoxical headaches may occur only after you have completed your tasks and expect to relax and enjoy some recovery time.

The Rebound Effect

The reason for this paradoxical migraine pattern is the "rebound" nature of these headaches. With this headache pattern, the fight-or-flight physiological events that accompany stress don't directly produce a headache, but instead set the stage for a future headache. This preheadache stress phase is associated with the increased release of a number of stress neurohormones that may stimulate sympathetic nervous system activation and lead to vasoconstriction of sensitive blood vessels. This vasoconstriction, in turn, can produce localized ischemia (inadequate blood supply) in the brain of susceptible individuals, leading to the initial aura (warning signs) of a forthcoming headache. The ischemic activity will also stimulate homeostatic counterregulatory neuroendocrine activity in an effort to increase blood flow to the constricted arteries.

Unfortunately, once the stress is over and you have the opportunity to relax, this counterregulatory effort may be so powerful that it overshoots the mark, causing the opposite vascular response, namely, overdilation. Along with the swelling of the overdilated artery comes the paradoxical "relaxation" headache.

Given this set of circumstances, the goal of self-regulation training must be to stabilize these vascular extremes by controlling the initial stress-related vasoconstrictive response and its associated neurochemical imbalance. Much as with tension headaches, you must learn to recognize the early cognitive and physiological signs of stress, and then try to "relax away" the muscle tension and characteristic autonomic nervous system (ANS) activation, which can set the stage for a later rebound headache. Thus, self-monitoring and using relaxation as a coping response is critical before the second more painful stage of the headache begins. However, once the painful overdilation phase has been reached, it might be too late for you to intervene with a self-control strategy. Your relaxation efforts can still help you remain calm while you wait for the pain to run its natural course or ease it with medication.

Stress as a Warning Sign

For some people, muscle tension of the upper back and neck may irritate nerves and blood vessels and trigger neurologic and vascular spasticity, thus initiating a migraine. In such cases, the tightness of the upper back and neck muscles also serves as a sign that it's time to try to relax away the muscle tension and hopefully to prevent the onset of the headache. Cold, clammy hands can also alert you to the fact that your sympathetic nervous system is overcharged. Employing the (BMW)I formula on such a day to the point of hand warming as frequently as possible may prevent tomorrow's headache. What you're trying to do is smooth out the neurophysiological events that can lead to a rebound headache.

Sleep Onset Headaches

Vascular rebound headaches are notorious for interrupting a good night's sleep, or greeting you when you wake up in the morning. It's particularly difficult to initiate any preventive action, whether through drugs or self-regulating, if you're sound asleep until the moment the pain strikes. But you can still take some preventive action here. If it's a time of month when you're prone to headaches, or if you feel emotionally or physically stressed as you lie down in bed, remember to do your (BMW)I relaxation exercise as you drift off to sleep. When you're feeling quite comfortable, focus your attention on an inner voice that says, "I will have a good night's sleep, pleasant dreams, and wake up feeling renewed." Of course, these need not be your exact words, but you get the idea.

While we're asleep, our minds seem to sort out the events of the day, possibly as part of moving them into long-term memory storage. These events seem to reactivate old memory "tapes" in the brain, tapes that can influence the content of our dreams and our physiological reactions. We hope that if the last tape in the mind's active consciousness is a "good night, sweet dreams, no headache" tape, that it will get the most play during the night. I didn't believe in the effectiveness of this self-regulation trick until several patients told me how well it worked for them. Try it. You certainly have nothing to lose.

Once a full-blown migraine attack is underway, it's too late to stop the headache in its tracks with self-regulation techniques. At this point you must do whatever you can do with medication, a quiet, dark room, cool washcloths, etc. Follow your (BMW)I formula to keep yourself relaxed and get your mind and body to work with the medications and cold cloths. Try working with some of the painkilling scripts presented above. Anything you can do to ride out the headache in a peaceful state will make the pain more tolerable and may even shorten the length of the episode.

Nonaura Migraine

The rationale and intervention strategies for nonaura migraines are quite similar to those of tension headaches and migraines with aura. Because the migraine without aura may reach full-strength very rapidly, or be already present when you wake up, catching it early and countering it with a relaxation response can be very difficult. For people facing this predicament, the best thing to do is try to self-monitor subjective tension levels throughout the day, especially on busy or stress-filled days, or for that matter in any situation that has led to a headache in the past. Try to take occasional relaxation breaks. In this way you may be able to reduce the upswing of stress-related neurochemicals that may later trigger a sudden rebound headache with little warning.

Posttraumatic Headaches

These are headaches that follow an injury to the head or neck. Since an injury can be the source of the same muscular and neuroendocrine mechanisms that are involved with other headaches, often posttraumatic headaches can be influenced by similar self-regulation strategies. However, the EMG biofeedback and physical strategies covered in chapter 7 are especially useful adjuncts with headaches that are caused by neck injuries.

Whiplash Headaches

One of the more common posttraumatic headaches is the headache that follows a whiplash-type injury to the muscles, tendons, and ligaments of the neck. Pain is also common where these neck structures attach to the base of the skull and to the bones of the spine and shoulders. Chronic discomfort following such an injury may also lead to less physical activity, which can result in a loss of muscular physical fitness. This muscular deconditioning, in turn, makes the muscles more vulnerable to the spasms and fatigue that can produce an aching headache. Thus, a vicious cycle is established linking pain, inactivity, and spasm, to even greater pain. Fortunately, general relaxation training and mental imagery may speed the effects of therapeutic exercises and counteract this cycle. Furthermore, muscle (EMG) biofeedback during these exercises can foster efficient and posturally correct use of painful muscles and joints.

Menstrual Headache

These are usually variations of vascular headaches, so there's little to add beyond what has been previously described. It's particularly important with these seemingly neurohormonal-driven headaches not to allow yourself to become fatalistic. This is a particularly important time of the month to monitor stress, to initiate relaxation, and to watch your diet and your medications very carefully. It's possible that hormone levels cause a temporary increased sensitivity to headache triggers, but by recognizing the triggers you might still be able to take some form of evasive action. Certain foods and especially alcohol may be more of a problem for these two or three days a month. The same may be true for stress.

Cluster Headaches

The menstrual headache message applies to cluster headaches as well. Cluster headaches are also variants of migraine vascular headaches. I have no special insight into what to do for this particularly troublesome headache pattern, other than to say that all you can do is to consider a cluster barrage as a time of extreme sensitivity to headache triggers. Simply do any and everything you possibly can to cope.

Furthermore, I encourage you to stay motivated to learn self-regulation techniques. The motivation to learn and practice self-regulation skills might not be very strong over the long stretches of time between outbreaks of the cluster headache. Too often, people come to a therapist for self-regulation training in the middle of a cluster sequence. But that's a difficult time to focus your attention on learning new self-management skills. The long stretches of headache-free time *between* the cluster outbreaks is when the skills must be introduced and developed. Then, using self-regulating strategies with medication during an outbreak may lessen the severity of the attack.

Sinus Headache

As you learned in chapter 2, many headaches that are labeled sinus headaches may not be true sinus headaches but rather vascular headaches involving blood vessels in or near the sinuses. It's also possible that conventional tension or vascular headaches in some cases might be triggered by increased sinus pressure. Don't assume that because you have a "sinus headache" that there's nothing you can do with self-regulation. Try your (BMW)I formula with intensified imagery. Even if you must seek treatment for a sinus infection, the self-regulation may make your ordeal more tolerable.

Behavioral Reminders and Tips

1. Try to keep a regular schedule. As much as is feasible, eat, sleep, and wake at the same time every day. This can increase the stability of the neurochemistry of your brain functions.

2. Be alert to common headache triggers, such as caffeine, alcohol, and foods containing monosodium glutamate. Caffeine intake needs special atten-

tion because although your morning cup(s) of coffee may prevent your caffeine withdrawal and morning headache, not drinking your morning coffee may trigger an afternoon headache.

3. Get up and stretch and move about periodically. This reduces muscle tension and cramping, encourages deep breathing, and may help to maintain stable brain chemistry.

4. Be alert to the possibility that both over-the-counter and prescription pain medications may contribute to the development of chronic headaches, even if they provide temporary relief.

5. Apply ice and/or heat to the headache site. Find out which can make a difference for you.

6. Massage your temples. While focusing on slow-deep breathing, place your fingertips on your temples and rub in a circular motion. This form of counterstimulation can promote relaxation.

7. Try acupressure stimulation. Rub the weblike space of your hand (where the bones of your thumb and forefinger come together in a V) with the fingers of your opposite hand or with ice wrapped in a washcloth. Rub your right hand if the left side of your head is hurting, and rub your left hand if the right side of your head hurts. See figure 5.1.

Chart Your Progress

As mentioned in chapter 3, the best way to measure pain is a simple ten-point rating scale. Keep a diary of your headaches and your stress levels. Whenever you have a headache, note how long it lasted and give the pain a rating. Rate the headache pain before and after a self-regulation session. Can you ease the pain at all? (See figures 5.2 and 5.3.)

The sample logs include examples of a daily and a weekly headache journal. From these samples you can put together your own log. Record those items that seem most relevant for you. Even on the days you don't have a headache, it can be useful to rate your mood (or subjective tension) and stress level for that day. Keeping such ratings for weeks, and even for months, can reveal trends and possible relationships that you might otherwise never recognize. For example, you might discover that your headaches tend to occur only after several days of heightened stressor levels. The logging process itself can alert you to those days that may require extra (BMW)I effort. The logs might also help you to evaluate whether over time

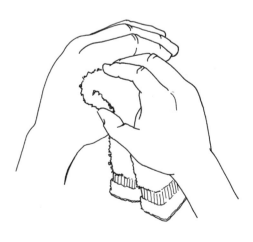

Acupressure Stimulation for Headaches

Figure 5.1:   (Ice wrapped in a washcloth)

Daily Headache Record

Symptom list:

Throbbing or pulsating pain _____	Dull and aching pain _____
Feeling of tightness and pressure _____	Nausea _____
Vomiting _____	Visual disturbance _____
Light sensitivity _____	Dizziness _____
Sharp pain _____	

	6	7	8	9	10	11	12	1	2	3	4	5	6	7	8	9	10	11	12	1	2	3	4	5	6
10																									
9																									
8																									
7																									
6																									
5																									
4																									
3																									
2																									
1																									
0																									

AM   NOON   MIDNIGHT   AM

0	**No pain**	
1–2	**Slight pain**—of which I am aware only when I think about it.	
3–4	**Mild pain**—but I can ignore it most of the time.	
5–6	**Moderate pain**—cannot be ignored, but I can still continue with all my normal activities.	
7–8	**Severe pain**—makes concentration difficult, but I can still manage tasks that are not too difficult.	
9–10	**Intense, incapacitating pain**—it is nearly impossible for me to do anything with this much pain.	

Medication: Each time headache medication taken list amount, type, and dosage level.

Notes:

_____   _____   _____

_____   _____   _____

_____   _____   _____

Figure 5.2

Weekly Headache Pain Journal

Name: _____   Date: _____

Each day pick a number between 0 and 10 to rate your headache pain level, mood type, activity restriction, and stressor level. Also list the number of minutes you practice self-regulation each day and the amount of medication taken.

Date	Headache level 0 is no pain 10 is pain as bad as it could be	Mood Type 0 is very good 10 is mood as bad as it could be	Activity Restriction 0 is no restriction 10 is unable to do anything	Stressor Level 0 is very low 10 is extremely high-stress day	Self-Regulation Number of minutes	Names of headache medications	Amount of each medication today	Possible triggers	Notes
	___ Severity ___ Time (a) ___ Duration (b)	___ Before HA ___ During HA	___ Before HA ___ During HA						
	___ Severity ___ Time (a) ___ Duration (b)	___ Before HA ___ During HA	___ Before HA ___ During HA						
	___ Severity ___ Time (a) ___ Duration (b)	___ Before HA ___ During HA	___ Before HA ___ During HA						
	___ Severity ___ Time (a) ___ Duration (b)	___ Before HA ___ During HA	___ Before HA ___ During HA						
	___ Severity ___ Time (a) ___ Duration (b)	___ Before HA ___ During HA	___ Before HA ___ During HA						
	___ Severity ___ Time (a) ___ Duration (b)	___ Before HA ___ During HA	___ Before HA ___ During HA						
	___ Severity ___ Time (a) ___ Duration (b)	___ Before HA ___ During HA	___ Before HA ___ During HA						

(a) time started and ended
(b) length of headache

Pain Severity Scale

0———1———2———3———4———5———6———7———8———9———10

No pain   Moderate pain   Worst pain can be

Figure 5.3

you're beginning to experience less subjective stress, even if your headache frequency and intensity have yet to change. Such information can give you reason to hope that your headache pattern will begin to change in time.

Scales to Monitor Thoughts That Disrupt Focused Attention

You may find your focusing efforts are disrupted by all types of random thoughts. The thoughts may not be particularly stressful but simply reflect your difficulty in keeping your attention focused. The key to dealing with this problem is not to "fight" the competing thought, but rather to train yourself to use it as a cue so that your attention can passively drift back to your primary focus of attention.

Competing Thoughts Scale

Fill out the brief competing thoughts scale below after each self-regulation practice session to chart your progress in focusing your attention.

_____ The level of competing, but nonstressful thoughts, I experienced during my self-regulation session.

_____ The level of competing, *mildly stressful* thoughts, I experienced during my self-regulation session.

_____ The level of competing, *highly stressful* thoughts, I experienced during my self-regulation session.

_____ My *overall level* of competing thoughts during my self-regulation session.

Rating Key

0 = Very few competing thoughts

1 = Slight occurrence of competing thoughts, but could refocus easily

2 = Moderate occurrence of competing thoughts, but could still refocus

3 = Many competing thoughts and a lot of difficulty staying focused, but could still reach a state of partial relaxation

4 = Almost constant competing thoughts, so I was unable to bring on feeling of relaxation

If you wish, list your major competing thoughts below.

_____

_____

_____

_____

_____

Intrusive Thoughts—The Impact of Events Scale (IES)*

If you find that much of the time, not just during self-regulation practice, you seem to be interrupted or preoccupied by disruptive, stressful thoughts about traumatic events in your life, you may wish to use the IES scale below. (Horowitz, Wilmer, Alvarez, 1979) This scale can help you evaluate whether you are making progress in controlling disruptive thoughts and feelings. Complete the scale now and then again after you practice self-regulation for several weeks. Check to see whether you have lowered your intrusive thoughts score.

Below is a list of comments made by people about stressful life events and the context surrounding those events. Read each item and decide how frequently each item was true for you during the past seven days, both for the event and its context. If the item didn't occur during the past seven days, choose the "Not at all" option. Indicate on the line at the left of each comment the number that best describes that item. You can then add up your total score.

_____ 1. I thought about it when I didn't mean to.

_____ 2. I had trouble falling asleep or staying asleep because of pictures or thoughts that came into my mind.

_____ 3. I had waves of strong feelings about it.

_____ 4. I had dreams about it.

_____ 5. Pictures about it popped into my mind.

_____ 6. Other things kept making me think about it.

_____ 7. Any reminder brought back feelings about it.

Rating Key

0 = Not at all

1 = Rarely

3 = Sometimes

5 = Often

A total of 4 or less would be considered a low score, 5–10 a medium score, and 11 or more a high score.

List stressful life event(s):

_____

_____

_____

_____

_____

* (used with permission of Mardi J. Horowitz)

Working with Cassette Tapes and a Therapist

Cassette tapes can be especially helpful early in the process of self-regulation. You can make your own tapes by reading from the scripts presented here, develop your own versions using these general ideas, or use commercially available tapes.

Ultimately, self-regulating is something you do yourself, even if a therapist helps you to develop your skills. Obviously, a therapist knowledgeable about headaches and self-regulation techniques can provide useful assistance, particularly if your headache pattern is severe. A therapist can respond to unique problems and make adjustments in a way that is impossible using a book or tape alone. And, of course, a therapist can provide the sometimes essential ingredient of encouragement that must come entirely from yourself if you are working with a book alone. Therapists who specialize in self-regulation training are most often psychologists or counselors. They may also be physical therapists, nurses, or occasionally physicians.

Be Patient and Develop a Positive Attitude

Headaches can be very frustrating because pain rapidly may become incapacitating and very difficult to control. Self-regulating is much easier with a mild tension headache than with a severe migraine but, remember, that absolutely anything you can do, even temporarily, is a moral victory. Any reduction in the frequency of headaches or the fading of pain in the throes of a headache is a sign that you're on the right track.

Even your feeling that you're less upset by the headache is a move in the right direction.

Don't set your immediate goals too high. If you feel you must get rid of your headaches right now, you might too easily become discouraged. Remember, you're trying to modify a very well habituated set of psychophysiological diatheses and triggers. Even if you are able to rapidly achieve control of breathing, muscle relaxation, and hand warming, this doesn't mean that you won't have any more headaches. You're trying to use these skills to counteract what may be a very complex and rigid neurophysiological response pattern leading to headaches.

See if you can turn self-management regulation into an interesting intellectual game for yourself. Become curious about your brain/body connections. Anything and everything you might notice is potentially useful. Can you make your arms feel as if they have become detached from your body? Remind yourself why this can happen. Can you feel your headache pain fade even a little as you focus on an imaginary contrasting, pleasurable image or sensation? Again, remind yourself of why this can happen. Be curious about why your hands do or do not get warmer on a given day.

The more interested you are, the more motivated you'll be to practice, and the more fun it'll be to try. That's why I believe that understanding the neurophysiological information contained in chapters 2 and 4 can make you better at self-regulating. Practicing even when you don't have a headache will increase your understanding and further motivate you. Cultivate a sense of how the mind/body connection works when you're not under the pressure of trying to cope with a headache. Then, start to develop some confidence in your ability to use this connection when you need it the most.

It's easy to feel discouraged in the midst of a painful headache attack unless you hold fast to the belief that in spite of your current pain, tomorrow will be a better day. If the overall frequency of your headaches this month is less than last month, and if your headache log reveals that the average intensity of your headaches has gradually been declining for several months, rest assured that you're doing something right. And, if you continue to practice the relaxation exercises daily, you can continue to expect your headache pattern to improve long after your first few weeks of attempting self-regulation techniques have passed.

Even when headaches are not primarily stress related, the ability to relax at will is useful. No matter what the cause of a headache, almost everyone finds the pain more tolerable when both the body and the mind are as relaxed as possible.

<u>Script</u>: Slow-Deep Breathing

Move your attention to your breathing. Make sure you are breathing comfortably, slowly, and with the movement of air visible in your stomach/abdomen. If helpful, count 1–2 for the inhalation and 3–4 for the exhalation. Let it become automatic, just feel the pleasant, healthful, slight rising and falling of your abdomen as your body breathes itself. With each quiet breath, let more and more tension leave your body. Notice the feelings of comfort and ease that come with each breath. If helpful, imagine you can watch the air leaving your body, like the water vapor you can see yourself exhaling on a cold day. Just watch the tension floating away as each cleansing breath provides ever more relaxation.

<u>Script</u>: Muscle Relaxation

Now that your breathing is settled into a really comfortable, easy in-and-out routine, move your attention to your jaw muscles. How do they feel? Let all the tension out of jaw; your mouth can be closed, but your teeth should not touch. Let the feeling of relaxation spread to where the muscle extends up to the top of your head, around your eyes and forehead, over to the back of your neck, around the sides of your neck to your throat. Imagine these muscles becoming as soft as if they were Jell-O, Play-Do, or sponge rubber. Let the feeling of relaxation flow down from your neck into your shoulder, right through the joints of your shoulders into your arms. Feel it moving down toward your elbows and into your forearms. It may help to imagine seeing the relaxation spread down from your neck into your arms and into your chest the way an ink stain would spread through tissue paper. Note the feeling of relaxed heaviness in your arms and the other parts of your body, as with each breath more muscle fibers exchange their tension for total, quiet, calm relaxation. You may want to make mental contact with your arms and hands and say in your mind, "Heaviness is flowing into my arms, warmth and heaviness are flowing into my hands." Let the flow continue through your lower abdomen, into your pelvic muscles and down your legs all the way to your feet. If one or both of your arms or legs or if your body feels almost disconnected and ready to float away, that's fine—it demonstrates how totally relaxed that part has become, and how little information it is sending to your brain. It is even letting your brain relax, almost as if you were asleep.

* Script: Hand Warming

Return your mental contact to your hands. Again say to yourself several times, "Heaviness and warmth are flowing into my hands." As you say this, feel the warmth, note that in your palms and especially in your fingers there may be a slight tingling, maybe even a faint hint of a pulse as the blood vessels in this highly sensitive part of your hands begin to expand ever so slightly. Don't be concerned if your hands do not actually seem warmer; just allow yourself to imagine what warmth feels like—heat, warmth; and comfort. What would it feel like to bathe your hands in warm water, or to rest them in the sun? You may want to imagine that it is a perfect day at the beach and, even if a cool breeze is blowing, you can feel the warmth of the sun on your skin.

Mental Imagery

Imagery has already been used extensively with the (BMW)I scripts. You can embellish these with your own additional imagery as much as you wish.

Key Word Summary

To ensure that you have thoroughly mastered the material in this chapter, write the definition of each term below in your own words.

Fading imagery: ____

____

____

Counterstimulation or competition imagery: ______________________

____

____

Symbolic imagery: ____

____

____

Distraction imagery: ____

____

____

Sleep onset headache: _____

_____

_____

Further Reading

Bakal, D. A. 1982. *The Psychobiology of Chronic Headache*. New York: Springer Publishing Company.

Catalano, E. M. 1990. *Getting to Sleep*. Oakland, CA: New Harbinger Publications.

Duckro, P. N., W. D. Richardson, and J. E. Marshall. 1995. *Taking Control of Your Headaches*. New York: Guilford Press.

Horowitz, M. J., N. Wilmer, and W. Alvarez. 1979. Impact of Event Scale: A Measure of Subjective Distress. *Psychosomatic Medicine, 41,* 209–218.

Rapoport, A. M. and F. D. Sheftell. 1990. *Headache Relief*. New York: Simon & Schuster.

CHAPTER 6

Physical Therapy and Exercise for Headaches

Susan J. Middaugh, P.T., Ph.D.

▲ Changing your posture

▲ Posture aids

▲ Therapeutic modalities

▲ Home exercise program

There is a set of physical problems that are commonly seen in people who have frequent headaches. They are as follows:

1. Poor posture of the head and upper back

2. Tight muscles with restricted range-of-motion of the neck

3. Irritable muscles that overreact when they are used and are slow to relax

4. Muscle pain with point tenderness

These musculoskeletal problems are interrelated and constantly reinforce each other. As a result, they tend to worsen over time. They are often found in people who have vascular as well as tension headaches, and are commonly thought to play an important (but not clearly understood) role in the development and continuation of headaches over time. This position is supported by the considerable success of treatment procedures designed to correct these four problems, including the therapies presented in this chapter.

The first part of this chapter covers posture, providing practical and straightforward methods to evaluate and correct common posture problems associated with headaches. The emphasis is on forward head posture, which overloads the muscles at the back of the neck and interferes with the smooth operation of the joints to which these muscles attach.

Then, in "Therapeutic Modalities," we introduce three simple and effective therapies—heat, ice, and vibration massage—for use at home or at work to counter headaches. Instructions are provided for the use of these self-administered modalities as part of a headache intervention program.

The rest of the chapter presents a home exercise program designed specifically for headaches. These exercises stretch overused muscles that have become tight, irritable, and hard to relax. The exercises also strengthen underused muscles that have become weak and overly lengthened. As muscle flexibility, strength, and relaxation increase due to these exercises, muscle pain and point tenderness typically decrease. The exercises also provide the basis for comfortable, good posture.

It's important to keep in mind that the therapies presented in this chapter aren't intended to stand alone. They're designed to complement the behavioral and medical therapies presented in this workbook to provide a maximally effective headache treatment program. The rationale for each therapy is provided in the sections below. Additional reading and primary references can be found at the end of the chapter.

Posture

This section presents simple and effective methods to evaluate and correct posture problems that may be contributing to your headaches. The posture shown in figure 6.1 is very common in people who have pain in the upper back, neck, or head, including headache and *temporomandibular joint* (TMJ or jaw) pain. The upper back is slumped, the shoulders are rounded, and the head is thrust forward. This head position, forward of the body's center of gravity, forces the muscles at the back of the neck to constantly contract. In addition, this head position increases the workload of these muscles, and the joints to which they attach, during head movements. This forward head posture can play a considerable role in the development of muscle pain and headache. Correcting this faulty posture, often produces a welcome reduction in headache symptoms.

Improving your posture can take some time and attention, but it's not difficult to do. Use the exercise program that's presented later to stretch out your tight muscles and strengthen your weak ones so that your body can comfortably assume a good position. Follow the methods described next to evaluate and change your posture habits. You can use inexpensive posture aids as illustrated in this section to support your body in good positions while sitting during the day and as you sleep at night. By making these efforts, good posture can become a comfortable new habit for you.

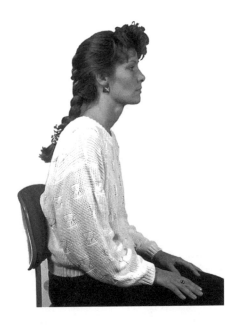

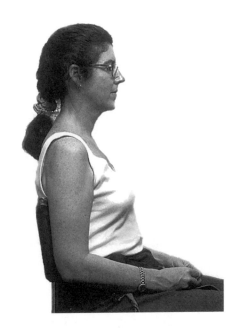

Figure 6.1: **The Forward Head Posture**   Figure 6.2: **Good Sitting Posture**

Checking and Changing Posture

Notice your posture as you sit, stand, walk, and work throughout the day. The following information will help you to identify problem areas and to make needed changes. It's important to keep in mind that good posture cannot be forced, military style. Good posture is largely a matter of balance and normally requires very little muscular effort.

Good sitting posture. Compare the forward head posture in figure 6.1 with the good sitting posture shown in figure 6.2. The back is now supported by a chair that provides good lumbar (low back) support. The shoulders are back. The head is straight, the ear is in line with the tip of the shoulder, and the chin is level. The elbow is touching the back of the chair. Each time you sit down, sit back in the chair. Let the chair support your back, and relax your shoulders. Slide your arms back until your elbows are touching the back of the chair. Your head should be up and balanced in place, not forced. If the chair provides correct support for the natural lumbar curve of your spine, your shoulders will automatically fall into the correct position when they are relaxed. Good lumbar support will also improve the position of your cervical spine and make it relatively easy to balance your head straight up and over your body's center of gravity (the midline of your trunk). If your chair doesn't provide this kind of support, it's essential to use a lumbar support aid, as shown later in this section.

Notice the position of your head and your elbows as you sit. If you hang your head forward, rather than balancing it upright, the weight of your head will pull your shoulders and upper back forward as well. If your elbows are in front of the midline of your trunk, the weight of your arms will pull your shoulders, upper back, and head forward. The head and arms each weigh 7 percent to 8 percent of body weight; for example, 8 percent = 12 pounds for a 150-pound person, and the total for one head plus two arms would be 36 pounds. This means that inevitably gravity will pull you into a slumped posture unless your head and elbows are lined up with the midline of your trunk. Use the turtle exercise shown in figure 6.3 to learn how to balance your head in a good position. Check your elbows often; they should be very close to the back of the chair.

The turtle exercise. See figure 6.3. This exercise can help you locate and practice good head alignment. Start in a good, basic sitting position as described above. Keep looking straight ahead and slowly push your chin forward, moving into an exaggerated forward head posture. Now, slowly pull your head back, keeping your chin level (do *not* tilt it upwards). Keep going back, little by little, until you find the point at which your head position starts to feel forced and uncomfortable. Ease up a little and let your head rest in that position, as far back as possible, but without feeling forced. Repeat this exercise. Do it once or twice a day, three to five repetitions each time, until you can easily find this balance point. As your flexibility improves with the exercise program presented later, you'll be able to balance your head a little farther back. Practice balancing your head in this upright position as you sit, stand, and walk. Try placing your fingers on the back of your neck, high up, at the base of your skull. Feel your neck muscles contract as your head moves forward, and relax as your head moves back to the balance point.

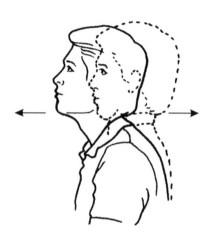

Figure 6.3: **The Turtle Exercise**

This is an excellent exercise to do with EMG biofeedback (electrodes placed at the base of the skull or over the masseter muscles, as explained in chapter 7).

Standing and walking posture. Stand with your head up and balanced, as described above, and your chin level. Relax your shoulders. If your head is up, then your shoulders will relax into a good position. If your head hangs forward, then your shoulders will follow. Now, observe your knees. People who have a forward head posture often stand with their knees locked. This locked-knee position pushes both the hips and the head forward. Loosen your knees and bend them slightly. Notice how this shifts your posture and makes it easier to keep your head in a good position. Check your head and your knees whenever you stand and learn to stand with your knees loose rather than locked. Check your head and shoulders when you walk. Notice whether you lean forward, hunch your shoulders, and look down at the ground while you are walking. Walk with your head up and your shoulders relaxed, even when you are in a hurry. (Don't worry, you can still see the ground.)

Working posture. Watch your posture at work and try to apply the principles of good posture (sitting, standing, and walking) given above. For example, make sure your office chair has good lumbar support, or use a lumbar support cushion. (See figure 6.4.) Notice your elbows and move your computer keyboard (or chair) closer so that you can work with your elbows at your side, rather than having to reach for the keyboard. Move your computer screen higher (or lower) so that you can see it with your head in a good position. Sometimes, the arrangement of a workstation and the requirements of specific work tasks can make it difficult to work in a good posture. If this is a problem, ask your doctor to refer you to an occupational therapist or a physical therapist specializing in workplace evaluation and ergonomics. This can be particularly helpful if your headaches are aggravated by work activities, such as operating a computer. Often a few inexpensive changes can make a large difference in your comfort during the day.

Posture aids

Lumbar support. Lumbar support is critical for good head posture. Cushions that are designed to fit the small of the back, such as the Posture Curve Lumbar Cushion from BodyCare, Inc., shown in figure 6.4, are effective, inexpensive, and available in many health product stores. One useful feature is a strap that can hold the cushion in the desired position against the back of the chair. Place the cushion in your chair or car seat and sit back. Let the chair and the cushion support your back. A rolled-up towel is a convenient alternative. Secure it at either end with a rubber band and place it in the small of your back. An airline pillow works well when flying. Airline seats and many recliners have rounded seat backs. Your lower spine rounds to match this configuration and your shoulders and head are then pushed forward. A lumbar support cushion, a rolled towel, or a small pillow placed in the small of the back will reestablish the normal curvature of

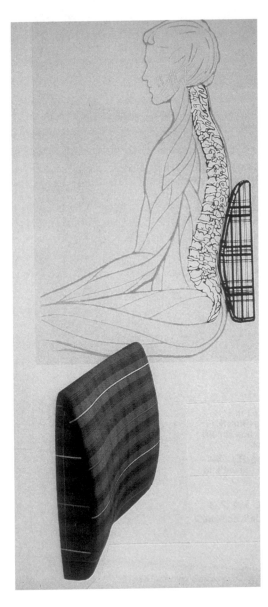

Figure 6.4: **The Posture Curve Lumbar Cushion**

your lower spine. This, in turn, will shift the position of your upper spine. Your shoulders and head will move back into a comfortable, upright position.

Footrests. Footrests are not designed to "rest" the feet but to position the legs when sitting. Many chair seats are not low enough to the floor to permit a correct leg position and this will affect the posture of the entire body. Observe the location of your knees. They should be slightly higher than your hips. If your knees are lower than your hips, then the weight of your legs will pull on your pelvis. This pull is transmitted to your low back, which will feel tight and uncomfortable. When this happens, the tendency is to lean forward in the chair to take the tension off the low back. One simple solution is to put a book or two on the floor to make a footrest that raises your feet and knees to the desired height (an old phone book works well). Now you can sit comfortably, all the way back in the chair, with your back correctly supported, and your head in a good posture.

Orthopedic pillow. An orthopedic pillow, such as the 4-in-1 WAL-PIL-O from the RoLoKe Co., shown in figure 6.5, can improve the position of your head during sleep. The WAL-PIL-O comes in several sizes and provides a choice of softer versus firmer support. It's very common for individuals with forward head posture to sleep with their head propped up on two or more pillows at night. This sleeping position places a continuous, eight- hour strain on the muscles of the neck and upper back and can be a major source of neck pain, and headache, the next morning. The pillow should provide good support under your neck, and should position your head in line with your trunk. Your head should not be angled upward. The same principles apply whether you sleep on your side or on your back. If your neck is tight, at first you may not be comfortable in a correct sleeping position. Start out each night using your new orthopedic pillow (or at least an improved arrangement of your old pillow). When you begin to be uncomfortable, shift back to your old method for the rest of the night. Gradually increase the time you spend in the improved sleeping position. This will become more comfortable as you make progress with the exercise program described later. Many individuals report a noticeable decrease in neck pain and headache once they are sleeping in a good position regularly. For some people, this change produces major improvement.

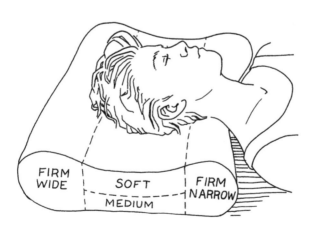

Figure 6.5:   The 4-in-1 WAL-PIL-O

Therapeutic Modalities

This section discusses three simple and effective self-administered therapies—heat, ice, and vibration massage—that can reduce the frequency and severity of headache symptoms when they're used as part of a comprehensive headache management program. All three therapies share a common feature: they can temporarily reduce your pain. The sensations of heat, cold, and vibration travel through many of the same nerve pathways as pain and are thought to *mask* or *block* the transmission of pain signals coming from the same area of the body. In addition, each of these three modalities has some unique features and uses. These are described below with instructions on how to use them effectively for headache management.

Heat

Use heat, applied to the muscles of your neck, *before* you exercise.

When you first begin the exercise program presented later, your muscles may become very sore, even with just a few repetitions of the gentlest neck exercises. This, in turn, can increase headache symptoms. *Most of this initial soreness can be circumvented by warming your neck muscles before exercising.* Heat increases the elasticity of muscles and connective tissue, increases local circulation, and increases muscle metabolism. As a result of applying heat, your muscles will stretch more easily, work more efficiently, and be less likely to become sore. Moist heat is particularly effective for this purpose. Following are two convenient methods for applying moist heat prior to exercise.

Warm showers. Take a warm shower and focus the flow of warm (not too hot) water on your neck and shoulder muscles for the final few minutes. You may be tempted to carry out your daily neck stretches (Exercises No. 2–No. 5 in the exercise program) while standing in the shower. This can be done on occasion as a shortcut but shouldn't be done on a regular basis. These neck stretches will be far more effective when you first warm your muscles for ten to fifteen minutes, and then sit down, with your back supported in a good posture, and your muscles relaxed, while you concentrate completely on slow, high-quality stretches.

Homemade microwave heat pack. Warm your neck muscles for ten to fifteen minutes before you exercise with the following easy-to-use, moist heat pack made from rice. Fill a long, fluffy athletic sock with uncooked rice. A knee-high tube sock works well. Tie a knot in the open end of the sock, or use rubber bands to serve as ties to close off a few inches at both ends. Place the rice-filled sock in the microwave oven and heat it on "high" for two to three minutes. Check the temperature to determine the best length of time to heat the rice in your microwave. Wrap the sock around your neck, lie down on your back or sit with your head supported, and allow your muscles to relax. This rice pack will mold easily to fit your neck (or other body areas) and will provide a comfortable moist heat for twenty to thirty minutes, which is the maximum length of time that heat should be applied at any one time. This is an excellent time to practice relaxation techniques and abdominal breathing. This rice pack is reusable: the same rice-filled sock can be reheated many times. Don't dampen the rice or the sock; the moisture will come from the natural water content of the uncooked rice. If you do not have a microwave you can use a heating pad. Models are widely available with a moist heat option.

Ice

Use ice, applied to the back of the neck, *immediately after you exercise to prevent sore, stiff muscles the following day.* Also use ice, applied to the back of your neck, to prevent headaches. Many people use ice, usually placed on the forehead, to reduce discomfort *after* a headache has started. However, ice can be far more effective when it is used *before* a headache develops, or at the earliest sign of a headache. Ice can be a very valuable addition to behavioral strategies for headache prevention and early intervention. These two uses of ice, for prevention of pain after exercise and prevention of headaches, are described below.

Multiple effects. Ice has multiple physiological effects that are useful in pain and headache control. These effects are achieved in ten to thirty minutes depending on (a) the method of ice administration and (b) the depth of the tissue involved. First, cold has a direct analgesic (painkilling) effect. It can slow nerve conduction and block nerve transmission to produce localized numbness and thus provide pain relief. In addition, cold can constrict blood vessels, both through the reflex actions of the sympathetic nervous system, and through direct cooling of the blood vessel walls. Cold also slows biochemical reactions and this can reduce tissue damage due to exercise and prevent delayed-onset pain. Finally, cold decreases the reflex response of the muscle to stretch and this can reduce the tendency of tight, painful neck muscles to overreact to movement. The beneficial effects of ice linger for several hours after the ice is removed, as the cooled tissues slowly rewarm to their previous temperature.

Easily applied. Ice can be applied easily by using inexpensive, reusable ice packs that are commercially available in the health products section of drug stores. Look for ice packs that stay soft and pliable when they're frozen. The Ace Brand Reusable Cold Compress™, for example, is inexpensive and widely available. It can be kept in the freezer compartment of a refrigerator (or a small beverage ice chest) at home or at work and will remain pliable when frozen. It's cloth covered and has a convenient shape (5 x 11 inches) that molds comfortably to the back of your neck and head. Single use, "shake and freeze" ice packs are also available. These don't require refrigeration and are convenient when traveling. One example is the Ace Brand Instant Cold Compress. Wrap your ice pack with a thin layer of towel, place it around the back of your neck, and lie down on your back for fifteen minutes. Let your muscles relax. If you can't lie down, sit with your head supported. A chair that is placed close enough to the wall to provide head support can work well. These small ice packs will retain the cold, at safe temperatures, for fifteen to twenty-five minutes. Another inexpensive and safe method is to use frozen peas in a plastic bag, wrapped in a towel, as an ice pack.

Caution: If you use a large ice pack or a bag of crushed ice, use more towel layers and don't leave it on longer than twenty-five minutes. Take the ice off sooner if the area goes numb. The deeper tissue will continue to cool even after the ice is removed, and the numb skin can become damaged if it remains in contact with the ice. This isn't a problem with smaller ice packs because they don't stay frozen long enough to pose a risk. If you're reluctant to use ice, or if you find ice uncomfortable at first, wrap the ice pack in several towel layers until it's just cool, not cold. Gradually reduce the layers of towel from day to day as you get used to the cold. Most people who are reluctant to use ice become enthusiastic users once they have tried it for a while and see how effective it can be.

Preventing pain after exercise. Ice can prevent the muscle pain and stiffness that typically occur after unaccustomed exercise. This use of ice is very familiar: a baseball pitcher will encase his pitching arm in ice immediately after a game, not because it hurts now (it usually doesn't), but because it's going to hurt and stiffen later (if ice isn't applied). This delayed-onset pain and stiffness can appear within a few hours, or as late as two days after the activity. When you begin the exercise program, use ice, placed at the back of your neck, immediately after you finish exercising. This will prevent stiff, sore muscles and an increased headache the following day. Once your muscles have become accustomed to these exercises, ice will no longer be needed. In the same way, use ice immediately after other activities that involve unaccustomed or extended use of your neck and shoulder muscles. For example, use ice after a game of tennis, after driving for long distances, or after any other physical activity that you suspect, based on your past experience, may produce neck pain or headache.

Preventing headaches. Ice can be very effective in preventing headaches. There are two complementary methods, and you should use both for full benefit. One method is to apply ice at the back of the neck, as described above, at the earliest sign of a headache. This can prevent the headache from developing further or reduce its severity and duration. Ice can also be timed to prevent a headache *before* it begins, if there's a predictable pattern of headache onset. An example of this is using ice in the early afternoon if headaches often develop around 3:00 p.m. This use of ice can be a valuable addition to the headache intervention strategies that are presented elsewhere in this workbook. The second method is to apply ice to the back of your neck once or twice a day on a regular basis, even on pain-free days. Some people with headaches have very little warning, or they haven't yet learned to recognize the warning signals that do occur. Others have essentially a constant headache that varies in intensity but doesn't start and stop. Many, if not most people, have frequent periods in which they overuse their neck and shoulder muscles in the course of everyday activities without realizing it. This can produce muscle fatigue and discomfort on the same day, as well as delayed-onset pain the following day. Under these conditions, the regular daily use of ice can be an effective prevention tool. Apply ice to the back of your neck at least once, and preferably twice, daily. Good times to do this are around noon (end of the morning or early afternoon) and 5:00 p.m. (end of the afternoon or early evening) for about fifteen minutes. This same quarter hour also can include deep relaxation, abdominal breathing, and other therapies.

Vibration Massage

Vibration and massage can be useful to reduce muscle pain and stiffness and aid muscle relaxation. There is a high incidence of muscle tenderness (variously termed point tenderness, tender point, or trigger point) in the muscles of the neck, shoulders, and upper back of individuals who have frequent headaches. These muscles are often tight, overreact to stretching, and are slow to relax after use. Although massage can be beneficial in managing these symptoms, it has the considerable disadvantage of requiring the services of another person. Vibrating muscle massagers, on the other hand, can be used without assistance, at little expense, as often as desired, at any time or place, with your clothes on. Furthermore, you control the intensity of the therapy when you do it yourself. Vibration has been shown to have a pain-relieving effect that compares very favorably with that of electrical stimulation (TENS), and this effect can last for several hours.

Vibrating muscle massagers. Long-handled, vibrating muscle massagers, such as the Panasonic Reach Easy Muscle Massager shown in figure 6.6, are inexpensive and widely available. The essential feature is a long handle (twelve to eighteen inches) that has an angle or a curve making it possible to reach your back muscles comfortably. A cordless and rechargeable model is very convenient and can be used outdoors, in the car, or at the office. Two levels of intensity (low and high) are usually standard and desirable. Avoid features that can substantially increase the weight (and cost) of this hand-held device and have no added therapeutic value. Prime examples are metal heads that heat up and multiple attachments with knobs and projections (these can bruise the muscle).

When you use this device, the muscles that are being massaged should stay relaxed. This means that the massager should be held in the *left* hand to massage

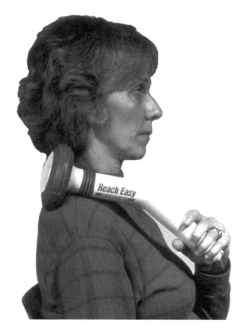

Figure 6.6:   **The Panasonic Reach Easy Muscle Massager**

the *right* shoulder muscles, as illustrated in figure 6.6. Begin on the low setting and explore your muscles for tender areas. These will be sensitive to the vibration as the massager passes over them. This is an excellent way to locate tender areas in your muscles. Common areas are the back of the neck, across the top of the shoulders, all around the shoulder blade, and down the back of the upper arm. Don't apply heavy pressure or leave the vibrating surface on one spot for minutes at a time. Instead, vibrate around and then lightly over each tender area for a minute or two, and repeat for the areas that need it the most. This vibration massage usually feels very good. If any area is too sensitive to touch, simply vibrate all around the sensitive area and don't vibrate directly over it. With regular use of vibration, the sensitivity of these tender areas usually will decrease over the course of several days. Massaging the muscles at bedtime, and again first thing in the morning, often reduces muscle symptoms that tend to develop over-night. To stay comfortable at home and work, massage your problem areas once or twice during the day.

A Home Exercise Program

This section presents an exercise program that is designed to systematically stretch, strengthen, and relax the muscles of the neck and shoulder girdle (the shoulder, upper back, and upper chest). As stated previously, if you have frequent headaches you'll often have a tight neck, weak upper back, and a forward head posture. In addition, many of the muscles in your neck and shoulder girdle will have tender points. These muscle problems are interrelated and are thought to play a major role in the development and maintenance of headaches. The follow-ing exercise program is designed to correct these muscle problems. It can be an effective addition to a headache treatment program.

Before You Start

Check with your doctor. Before beginning this, or any, exercise program, check it out with your doctor. He or she may refer you to a physical therapist to assist you in starting safely. If you've had any injuries or surgery involving your head, neck, back, or shoulders, these exercises should be supervised. Problem exercises should be modified or eliminated, and alternative exercises substituted, to meet your individual needs. This is particularly important for those who have current or past problems with a cervical disc, cervical instability, rotator cuff repair, shoulder dislocation, or fixed spinal deformities from degenerative joint disease or osteoporosis. Many people with headaches also have low back prob-lems. When this is the case, a more comprehensive exercise program may be needed.

Don't start all of these exercises at once. As with most exercise programs, this set of exercises begins with relatively easy exercises designed to stretch tight muscles. It then adds more difficult exercises designed to strengthen weak mus-cles. The initial exercises in this series prepare your muscles for the later, more advanced exercises, so it's important to do them in the order in which they are described, and to resist the temptation to skip some. Attempting to do too much too soon is a common mistake when starting a therapeutic exercise program. If you begin with ten repetitions of all eleven of these exercises on the first day, this can easily produce major problems with painful, stiff muscles and can also increase headache. You might come to the erroneous conclusion that "exercise just makes things worse." In contrast, the same eleven exercises can be very effective and relatively trouble-free if you begin with no more than three repetitions of the first few, make sure you do each one correctly, allow your body to get used to these new movements, and then gradually increase the repetitions. Follow the instructions that are provided to guide you.

Expect short-term soreness. When you begin these exercises, expect mild to moderate short-term soreness. The therapeutic modalities described earlier can prevent and minimize this initial soreness. All exercise movements should be carried out slowly and gently, without forcing the movements, and without jerking or bouncing. As you move, notice the sensations of stretching and moving in your muscles and joints and focus on letting your muscles relax as they stretch. You may have some mild discomfort while performing one or more of these exercises, but don't push to the point of actual pain. It's normal to have some muscle soreness the day after starting any new physical activity, but this should rapidly decrease over the course of two or three days as you continue doing the exercises. Most of this discomfort can be prevented by using heat on the muscles before exercising and applying ice to the same muscles after you exercise, as described earlier. If you have problems getting started on these exercises, stop and ask your physician to refer you to a physical therapist for supervision.

Cervical (Neck) Stretches

Exercises No. 1 through No. 5 are designed to stretch tight neck muscles and restore the normal flexibility and range-of-motion of the neck. When the neck muscles are too short and tight, normal head movements pull on these tight muscles all day long. To protect themselves, tight muscles respond by tensing up to resist being pulled when, instead, they should be relaxing to permit fluid movement. The result is strain on the muscles and the joints to which they attach, and this strain can become a source of pain and discomfort in the head and neck area.

For these five exercises, sit in a chair with good back support, keep your head straight, chin level, hands in your lap, and elbows touching the back of your chair as shown in figure 6.2. Begin with three slow repetitions of each exercise, performed once each day, for the first three days. Once the initial soreness is over, gradually increase to a maximum of five repetitions. Do these five exercises together, as a set, rather than scattered throughout the day. The muscles will increase in flexibility with each repetition and each exercise, for optimum effectiveness.

Exercise No. 1. Shoulder Shrug/Relax

This exercise will both relax and stretch the muscles that shrug the shoulders upward (upper trapezius and levator scapulae). See figure 6.7. Many people with

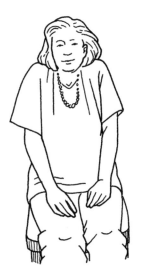
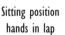
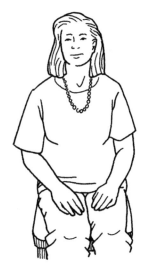

Sitting position
hands in lap

Figure 6.7:   **Exercise No. I. Shoulder Shrug/Relax**

headache, neck pain, or jaw pain go through the day with these muscles tense and their shoulders partially shrugged. Their neck muscles adapt to this habitual "tensed-up shoulders" position by becoming short, tight, and often painful. Once this happens, it can become difficult to relax these muscles because a normal position (shoulders relaxed down) now stretches these tight muscles, and this may be uncomfortable. In response, the muscles will tend to tense up again. This is an excellent exercise to do with EMG biofeedback (electrode placement over the upper trapezius at the shoulder).

Slowly and gently shrug your shoulders up toward your ears and notice what your muscles feel like as they tense. Hold your shoulders up for three seconds. Then relax slowly and let your shoulders down, little by little, until they're all the way down. Don't push or force your shoulders down; instead, let them relax down. Then, focus on leaving your shoulders relaxed for thirty seconds. Repeat. This exercise can be discontinued once you've learned to relax your shoulders easily and are comfortable in this relaxed position. This will typically occur at the time you're ready to begin Exercise No. 9.

Exercise No. 2. Cervical Rotation

This exercise will stretch tight muscles at the back and sides of the neck. See figure 6.8. Begin by looking straight ahead, with your shoulders relaxed. Slowly and gently turn your head to the right as if you were going to look over your shoulder. When you've gone as far as you can easily go, without forcing or pushing, hold this position for fifteen

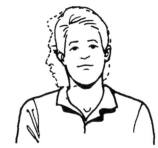

Figure 6.8:

Exercise No. 2. Cervical Rotation

seconds. Focus on relaxing the opposite (left) shoulder down, and let time and gravity gently stretch the left side of your neck. Return to the start position and relax. Now turn your head to the left, hold for fifteen seconds, and focus on relaxing the opposite (right) shoulder down. Return to the start position. Repeat.

Exercise No. 3. Cervical Flexion

This exercise will stretch tight muscles at the back of the neck. See figure 6.9. Begin by looking straight ahead, with your chin level and your shoulders relaxed.

1. Curl your chin down toward your chest and let your head relax forward. Hold for five seconds and focus on letting the muscles at the back of your neck relax and stretch. Don't force this exercise; just let time and the weight of your head produce a gentle stretch.

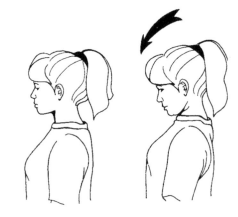

Figure 6.9:

Exercise No. 3. Cervical Flexion

2. Keep your head forward and gently turn your chin a little to the right. Hold for five seconds and focus on letting the muscles relax and stretch at the back of your neck on the left.

3. Keep your head forward and gently turn your chin a little to the left. Hold for five seconds and focus on the muscles at the back of your neck on the right. Return to the start position. Repeat.

Caution: If your neck is very tight and you feel a strong stretch in step 1, or have difficulty doing the chin movements in steps 2 and 3, then begin with step 1 only and hold this single position for fifteen seconds. Once your neck becomes a little looser (in a few days or a few weeks; take your time), add the chin movements to right and left. This combination of neck flexion and chin rotation can be difficult to do at first, but it's very effective in stretching any tight muscles at the base of your skull.

Exercise No. 4. Jawline Stretch

This exercise will stretch tight muscles at the front and along the sides of your neck (sternocleidomastoid, scalenes, and omohyoid). See figure 6.10. These muscles become short and tight if you have a forward head posture or an upper-chest breathing pattern. This exercise is particularly important if you have jaw (TMJ) symptoms, because these muscles affect both the resting position and the motion of your jaw.

Begin by looking straight ahead with your chin level and shoulders relaxed. Keep your lips closed.

1. Tilt your chin upward until you feel a stretch just under the chin and along the jawline. Hold for five seconds.

2. Keep your chin up and tilt your head a little to the right. The stretch will now be focused near the corner of your jaw on the left (near your ear and TMJ). Hold for five seconds.

3. Keep your chin up and tilt your head a little to the left. The stretch will now be focused near the corner of your jaw on the right. Hold for five seconds. Return to the start position. Repeat.

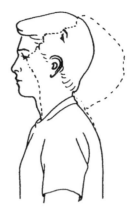

Figure 6.10:

**Exercise No. 4.
Jawline Stretch**

Caution: The object of this exercise is *not* to tilt the head back as far as possible (cervical extension), which can cause pain at the back of the neck. Instead, the purpose is to stretch under the jaw and along the jawline. This can be accomplished without tilting the chin up very high. Try pulling your head slightly back to a more upright position, as you did in the turtle exercise (see figure 6.3), to position your head a little better before you tilt your chin up. As with Exercise No. 3, at first you may have difficulty doing all three parts of this exercise. If so, begin with step 1 only and hold it for fifteen seconds. Add steps 2 and 3 later.

Suggestion: Once you've learned how to do Exercises Nos. 3 and 4, alternate them. Do one repetition of Exercise No. 3, followed by one repetition of Exercise No. 4. Continue alternating until you have completed the desired five repetitions for each exercise.

Exercise No. 5. Lateral Head Tilt

This exercise will stretch tight muscles at the side of the neck (scalenes and upper trapezius). See figure 6.11. These muscles rapidly become short and tight if you frequently tense your shoulders upward. This exercise is often omitted from stretching programs, but it's an important exercise for headache and jaw pain. Keep looking straight ahead (nose pointing forward), leave both of your shoulders relaxed and level, and tilt your right ear toward your right shoulder. Don't force your head to the right. Just relax and let gravity do the

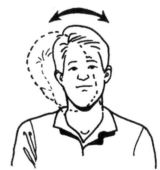

Figure 6.11:

Exercise No. 5. Lateral Head Tilt

work. The weight of your head as it tilts to the right will stretch the left side of your neck. Focus on relaxing the opposite (left) shoulder down. Don't let your whole body lean to the right, just your head. Hold for fifteen seconds. Return to the start position and relax. Now, tilt your head to the left, stretching the right side of your neck. Focus on relaxing the opposite (right) shoulder down. Hold for fifteen seconds. Return to the start position. Repeat, alternating right and left stretches.

Caution: Although this is a simple exercise to do, it's also easy to overdo. The lateral neck muscles are often very tight and the weight of the head (averaging 12 pounds) can generate a strong stretch on these tight muscles. Exercises No. 1 through No. 4 will partially stretch these same muscles and prepare them for this exercise. In addition, you can easily control the amount of stretching during this exercise. Just let your head tilt part way and hold at the point that produces a stretch, but not pain. Over time, as these muscles loosen, let your head tilt a little farther.

Shoulder Girdle Stretches

Once you've started Exercises No. 1 through No. 5, recovered from the initial soreness you may have experienced, and increased to five repetitions (usually one to two weeks), you're ready to add Exercises Nos. 6, 7, and 8. These will stretch the muscles of your shoulders, chest, and upper back. Individuals who have a forward head posture, rounded shoulders, and a shallow, upper-chest breathing pattern typically get tight throughout the shoulder girdle. It's necessary to stretch these areas to restore the muscle flexibility and strength that are needed for good posture and comfortable movement. These exercises should be carried out lying on your back, without a pillow, and on a firm surface, such as a carpeted floor or an exercise mat (not on a bed).

Exercise No. 6. Chest Wall Stretch

This exercise stretches the pectoral muscles, the rib cage, and the upper spine. See figure 6.12. Lie on your back, bend your knees, and put your feet flat on the floor. Place both of your arms in the position shown, with your arms out to the side, the elbows bent, and the back of your hands resting on the floor. Relax in this position and let time and gravity gently stretch your muscles and joints. If your hands don't touch the floor, don't force them down. Your hands will gradually move toward the floor as your shoulder muscles stretch out, over days. The goal is to lie in this position continuously for five minutes, once a day. Start with one or two minutes and notice where you feel the stretch—your shoulders, neck, chest, and upper back. Stop if this stretch increases to the point of pain, and notice how long this took. Repeat the next day. Gradually increase the time, day by day, until you reach a maximum of five minutes.

This exercise provides a good opportunity to evaluate your posture. How easily can you lie in this position? How far off the floor are your hands? If you're used to sleeping with your head propped up on two pillows, if your habitual head posture is very far forward, or if your upper back is quite rounded, you may need to start this exercise with a pillow under your head. As you stretch out, over days, gradually position your head closer to the floor. A person with good flexibility can easily lie in this position for five minutes and will feel a pleasant stretch in the upper back. If you don't even feel a stretch after five minutes, you can skip this exercise.

Lying on back, looking up toward ceiling, arms
on floor, palms up, shoulder 90° elbow 90°

Hands palm up

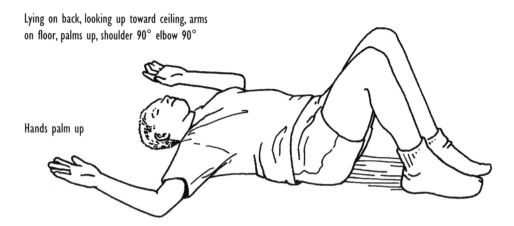

Figure 6.12:   Exercise No. 6. Chest Wall (Pectoral) Stretch

Suggestion: If your neck feels uncomfortable in this position, place a small rolled towel under the curve of your neck to provide support. If your tailbone becomes uncomfortable, place one ankle on top of the other knee, or put both legs up on a chair. Either strategy will tilt your pelvis, flatten the small of your back against the floor, and take the pressure off your tailbone.

Exercise No. 7. Shoulder Flexion

See figure 6.13. Lie flat on your back with your knees bent, feet flat on the floor, and your arms at your side. Raise both of your hands straight up toward the ceiling. Touch your thumbs together, keep your arms relatively straight, and keep going over your head until the your hands are as close to the floor as they will go without forcing. Hold for five seconds and focus on relaxing the muscles around your shoulders, while gravity stretches your arms a little closer to the

Starting with arms at side
raising arms up toward ceiling and over head

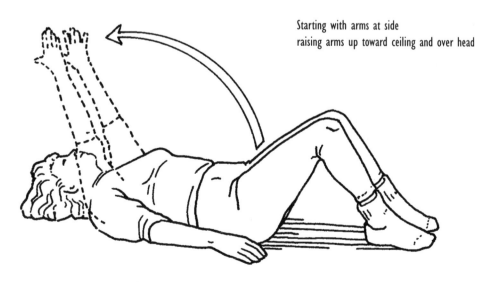

Figure 6.13:   Exercise No. 7. Shoulder Flexion

floor. Raise your arms back up and return to the start position. Repeat. As you gain flexibility (usually one to two weeks), you'll be able to easily rest the back of your hands on the floor over your head. Your elbows will be slightly bent but close to your head.

Exercise No. 8. Shoulder Abduction

See figure 6.14. Lie on your back with your knees bent, feet flat on the floor, your arms at your side, and your palms up. Keep your elbows relatively straight and slide the back of your hands along the floor, straight out to the side and up over your head. When you can no longer keep the back of your hands on the floor (do not force this exercise), just let your arms lift off the floor and keep going until your thumbs touch over your head. Hold for five seconds and let gravity gently pull your arms a little closer to the floor. Return to the start position. Repeat. As you gain flexibility, you'll be able to keep the backs of both hands on the floor until your thumbs touch over your head.

Do Exercises Nos. 7 and 8 daily. Begin with three repetitions for the first three days until you're over the initial soreness. Gradually increase by adding one repetition every other day to a maximum of ten repetitions each.

Shoulder Girdle Strengthening Exercises

Once you've started Exercises Nos. 6, 7, and 8, and have successfully increased to five minutes (No. 6) and ten repetitions (Nos. 7 and 8), and the backs of your hands can rest easily on the floor in the overhead position (two to three weeks), you're ready to add the final set of advanced exercises, Nos. 9, 10, and 11. These exercises will strengthen important postural muscles in your back that attach to your shoulder blade (the scapula) and the thoracic spine (paraspinal extensor muscles). These strengthening exercises can be done daily or every other day.

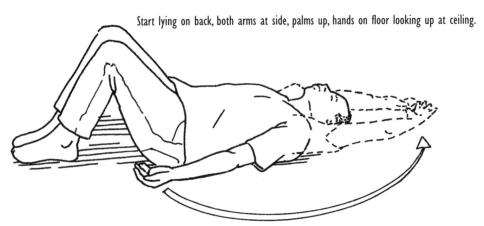

Start lying on back, both arms at side, palms up, hands on floor looking up at ceiling.

Scoot backs of hands out to the side on the floor until over head. End with backs of hands still on floor, palms up, thumbs touching or close.

Figure 6.14:   **Exercise No. 8. Shoulder Abduction**

Exercise No. 9. Scapular Stabilization

See figure 6.15. Lie on your back with your knees bent and feet flat on the floor. Start with a 1-pound weight in each hand (a 16-ounce can of fruit or a bottle of water works well) and your arms straight up toward the ceiling (position 1). Keep your elbows relatively straight (they'll be slightly bent) and lower your arms slowly until they're straight out to the side (position 2). Stop when the back of your hand is an inch *above* the floor and *don't rest your arm or hand on the floor.* Hold your arms just off the floor for three to five seconds and then return to position 1, which is the start position for this exercise. Repeat. Start with three repetitions for the first three days that you do this exercise and then gradually increase to five repetitions.

Once you've reached five repetitions of Exercise No. 9, add the same 1 pound weight to Exercise No. 7 above. Decrease Exercise No. 7 to five repetitions (the weight now makes it harder). When you reach the overhead position, hold the weights just off the floor for three to five seconds (thumbs toward the floor). Do Exercises Nos. 7 and 9 together and alternate sets of five repetitions each. That is, first do five repetitions of Exercise No. 7, and then do five repetitions of Exercise No. 9. When this becomes relatively easy, add a second set of five repetitions of Exercise No. 7 and later add a second set of five repetitions of Exercise No. 9. Gradually increase to a maximum of three sets of five repetitions (fifteen total repetitions) of each exercise. You don't need to increase the weight above 1 pound, since this is a good amount of weight at the end of a long arm. Depending on body size and strength, some individuals may increase to (but should not exceed) 2 or 3 pounds.

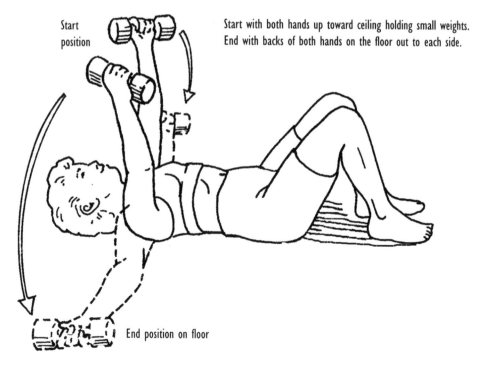

Start position

Start with both hands up toward ceiling holding small weights. End with backs of both hands on the floor out to each side.

End position on floor

Figure 6.15:   **Exercise No. 9. Scapular Stabilization**

It may seem unusual to exercise the muscles of the upper back while lying face up; however, you'll be able to feel these muscles contracting strongly in your back and between your shoulder blades as you do these two exercises with weights. This position (face up) also provides an excellent workout (stretch and strengthen) for two important muscles that lie between the rib cage and the shoulder blade and are particularly difficult to exercise (subscapularis and serratus anterior). This exercise also strengthens the muscles at the front of your neck (including the sternocleidomastoid). You may experience some initial soreness around your jawline and behind your ear when you start. As a bonus, tuck in your abdominal muscles to flatten and hold the small of your back against the floor (pelvic tilt) while you do these two exercises, and you'll also strengthen your abdominal muscles.

Exercise No. 10. Prone Hyperextension

See figure 6.16. Lie on the floor, face down (forehead touching the floor), with your arms resting on the floor straight out to the side at shoulder level. If your back is uncomfortable in this position, place a pillow under your waist.

1. First raise only your arms off the floor and *pinch your shoulder blades together.*

2. Hold this arm position while you gently lift your shoulders, forehead, and upper chest *a few inches* off the floor. Hold for three seconds and return to the start position, resting on the floor. Don't bend your neck backwards (keep looking at the floor) and *do not raise your legs.* These first two steps will strengthen your back muscles down to waist level. Begin with three repetitions for the first three days that you do this exercise, and then gradually increase to ten repetitions (two to four weeks or longer if needed).

   Once you're comfortable with ten repetitions, begin the advanced version by adding the next step.

3. Each time you lift your head and chest, also lift both legs *a few inches* off the floor. This will strengthen the muscles of your lower spine and hips as well. Reduce the repetitions from ten to five when you begin this advanced version, because you are now adding the weight of both legs. Gradually increase to a maximum of fifteen repetitions. This may take two to three months. If you have back problems, don't start this exercise without supervision.

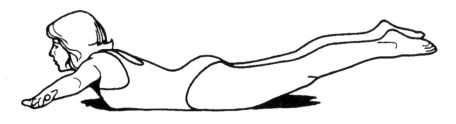

Figure 6.16:   **Exercise No. 10. Prone Hyperextension**

Exercise No. 11a. Wall Exercise

See figure 6.17a. Don't start this exercise unless the back of your hand can rest easily on the floor in Exercise No. 6 (see figure 6.12). Stand with your back against a wall, arms at your side, heels three to six inches away from the wall, knees bent slightly, and abdominal muscles tucked in to flatten the small of your back against the wall (pelvic tilt). Hold this pelvic tilt position as you slide the back of your fingers along the wall until your arms are straight out to your side at shoulder level. Bend your elbows to move your hands into the position shown in figure 6.17a. Hold this position, with your hand touching the wall, three to

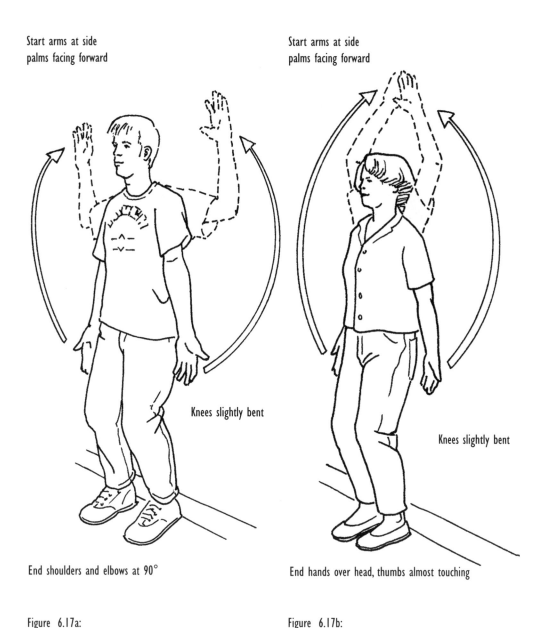

Start arms at side
palms facing forward

Start arms at side
palms facing forward

Knees slightly bent

Knees slightly bent

End shoulders and elbows at 90°

End hands over head, thumbs almost touching

Figure 6.17a:

Exercise No. 11a. Wall Exercise

Figure 6.17b:

Exercise No. 11b. Advanced Wall Exercise

five seconds. Return to the start position. Repeat. Start with three repetitions for the first three days that you do this exercise, and gradually increase to ten repetitions. When you're at ten repetitions, add Exercise No. 11b (below). If you don't have the flexibility that's needed for Exercise No. 11b, then stay with Exercise No. 11a and gradually increase to a total of fifteen repetitions.

Exercise No. 11b. Advanced Wall Exercise

See figure 6.17b. Don't start this exercise unless you can easily perform Exercise No. 8 (see figure 6.14). Once you start Exercise No. 11b you can stop Exercise No. 8, since both exercises include the same movement (shoulder abduction). Also, decrease Exercise No. 11a to five repetitions when you start Exercise No. 11b. Stand with your back against the wall in the same starting position as Exercise No. 11a. Hold the small of your back flat against the wall as you slide the back of your fingers along the wall, until your arms are straight out to your sides at shoulder level. Now, keep your elbows relatively straight (they will bend a little) and continue to slide the back of your fingers, still touching the wall, up over your head until your thumbs touch. You'll feel a strong contraction of your back muscles as your arms move overhead and your abdominal muscles will have to contract strongly to keep the small of your back against the wall. Hold this position for three to five seconds. Return to the start position. Repeat. Begin with three repetitions for the first three days that you do this exercise and gradually increase to five repetitions.

Do Exercises Nos. 11a and 11b together, alternating sets of five repetitions. That is, do five repetitions of No. 11a and then do five repetitions of No. 11b. When this becomes relatively easy, add a second set of five repetitions of Exercise No. 11a, and finally add a second set of five repetitions of Exercise No. 11b. This will provide a maximum of ten repetitions of each exercise.

Your Long Term Exercise Program

Exercise No. 1 can be discontinued once you have mastered basic shoulder relaxation and can leave your shoulders relaxed without discomfort, usually about the time you start Exercises Nos. 9, 10, and 11.

Exercises Nos. 2 through 5, the neck stretches, should be continued on a daily basis. You're likely to find that doing five slow repetitions of these stretches the first thing in the morning (perhaps after a warm shower) makes a large difference in how comfortably you go through the day. You may find it helpful to repeat these four exercises a second time, later in the day, if your neck stiffens up again. If increasing neck discomfort is one of your warning signs that a headache is developing, try doing three to five repetitions of these gentle neck stretches when this warning occurs, as part of your headache prevention strategy. *Do not stretch your neck constantly by doing one or two neck stretches all day long. This will not stretch the muscles, but will just jerk them around, and they'll react by tensing up.*

Exercise No. 11 should also be done on a daily basis. It's a wonderful posture exercise that both stretches and strengthens your muscles. Once you're used to this exercise, it'll feel very good, especially after sitting for a long period of time at a desk or computer. This exercise can be done in street clothes, without sweat, in the office, a hallway, or in a stairwell. Once you are adept at this exercise, it can be done with your back against a door frame, rather than a wall, when sufficient wall space is lacking.

Exercises Nos. 6, 7, 8, 9, and 10 all require getting down on the floor. These can be done every other day to build and then to maintain your strength and flexibility. Discontinue No. 8 if you're doing Exercise No. 11b.

Further Reading

Braun, B. 1991. "Postural differences between asymptomatic men and women and craniofacial pain patients." *Archives of Physical Medicine and Rehabilitation.* 72: 653–656.

Enwemeka, C., I. Bonet, J. Ingle, S. Prudhithumrong, F. Ogbahon, and N. Gbenedio. 1986. "Postural correction in persons with neck pain: Integrated electromyography of upper trapezius in three simulated neck positions." *The Journal of Orthopaedic and Sports Physical Therapy.* 8: 240–242.

Grandjean, E. 1988. *Fitting the Task to the Man: A Textbook of Occupational Ergonomics.* (4th ed.) London: Taylor & Francis.

Griegel-Morris, P., K. Larson, K. Mueller-Klaus, and C. A. Oatis. 1992. "Incidence of common postural abnormalities in the cervical, shoulder, and thoracic regions and their association with pain in two age groups of healthy subjects." *Physical Therapy.* 72: 425–431.

Guieu, R., M. Tardy-Gervet, and J. Roll. 1991. "Analgesic effects of vibration and transcutaneous electrical nerve stimulation applied separately and simultaneously to patients with chronic pain." *Canadian Journal of Neurological Sciences.* 18: 113–119.

Janda, V. 1988. "Muscles and cervicogenic pain syndromes." In *Physical Therapy of the Cervical and Thoracic Spine.* Edited by R. Grant. New York: Churchill Livingstone. 153–166.

Kee, W. G., S. J. Middaugh, and K. P. Pawlick. 1996. "Persistent pain in the older patient: Evaluation and treatment." In *Psychological Approaches to Pain Management: A Practitioner's Handbook.* Edited by R. J. Gatchel and D. C. Turk. New York: Guilford Publications, Inc. 371–402.

Kendall, F. P., E. K. McCreary, and P. G. Provance. 1993. *Muscles, Testing and Function: With Posture and Pain.* 4th ed. Baltimore: Williams and Wilkins.

Ku, Yu-Tsuan E., L. D. Montgomery, and B. W. Webbon. 1996. "Hemodynamic and thermal responses to head and neck cooling in men and women." *American Journal of Physical Medicine and Rehabilitation.* 75: 443–450.

Lundeberg, T., P. Abrahamsson, L. Bondesson, and E. Haker. 1988. "Effect of vibratory stimulation on experimental and clinical pain." *Scandinavian Journal of Rehabilitation Medicine.* 20: 149–159.

Mannheimer, J. S. 1994. "Prevention and restoration of abnormal upper quarter posture." In *New Concepts in Craniomandibular and Chronic Pain Management.* Edited by Harold Gelb. London: Mosby-Wolfe. 93–161.

Middaugh, S. J. 1989. "Biobehavioral Techniques." In *Physical Therapy.* Edited by R. Scully and M. Barnes. Philadelphia: J. B. Lippencott Co. 986–997.

Middaugh, S. and W. G. Kee. 1987. "Advances in electromyographic monitoring and biofeedback in treatment of chronic cervical and low back pain." In *Advances in Clinical Rehabilitation, Vol. I.* Edited by M. G. Eisenberg and R. C. Grzesiak. New York: Springer Publishing Co. 137–172.

Middaugh, S. J., W. G. Kee, and J. Nicholson. 1994. "Muscle overuse and posture as factors in the development and maintenance of chronic musculoskeletal pain." In *Psychological Vulnerability to Chronic Pain.* Edited by R. C. Grzesiak and D. S. Ciccone. New York: Springer Publishing Co. 55–88.

Pascarelli, E. D. and D. Quilter. 1994. *Repetitive Strain Disorder.* New York: John Wiley & Sons, Inc.

Scheetz, A. P. and D. E. Mathis. 1995. "Rice sock for pain and stress." *Postgraduate Medicine.* 98: No. 2, August, p. 118.

Travell, J. C. and D. G. Simons. 1983. *Myofascial Pain and Dysfunction: The Trigger Point Manual.* Baltimore: Williams and Wilkins.

Walpin, L. A. 1987. "The role of orthotic devices for managing neck disorders." *Physical Medicine and Rehabilitation: State of the Art Reviews,* Vol. 1, No. 1, February.

Whitney, S. L. 1989. "Physical agents: Heat and cold modalities." In *Physical Therapy.* Edited by R. M. Scully and M. R. Barnes. Philadelphia: J. B. Lippencott Co. 844–875.

CHAPTER 7

Biofeedback:
A Powerful Tool

▲ Defining biofeedback

▲ Combining biofeedback with (BMW)I

▲ Biofeedback for headaches

Biofeedback is a relatively new technology that first became popular in the 1970s. It has done much to stir up current interest in the process of self-regulation. Biofeedback has contributed to self-regulation behavioral techniques by making the process more objective and measurable and, therefore, more scientifically respectable.

Biofeedback

Biofeedback can be used in a wide variety of ways. Some applications of biofeedback overlap a great deal with other self-regulation techniques, although other applications are quite different. Thus, when a person says, "I did biofeedback training," "I had biofeedback," or "I practiced my biofeedback," such a statement tells us very little. Also, don't confuse the term biofeedback with the term *biorhythms*, which is short for biological rhythms. The two terms have no direct relationship. Biorhythms refer to the fact that much of our physiological functioning and behavior follow regular rhythms—our twenty-four-hour daily pattern of waking and sleep being the best example of such rhythms.

Definition

Biofeedback refers to any monitoring of physiological functions for the purpose of providing information that can be used to control (i.e., self-regulate) those functions. The goal is to use ongoing information about the status of the physiological function to increase, decrease, or stabilize that function. Thus, if you were to measure your pulse rate for fifteen seconds, then try to speed it up or slow it down, and then measure it again for another fifteen seconds, you would be engaging in a crude form of biofeedback.

The feedback, however, can be made much more precise by using electronic monitoring instruments. Heart rate feedback from the monitor can correspond to each individual heartbeat, rather than waiting for a fifteen-second average. The basic paradigm involves sensors, electronic amplifiers, computer processing of the signal, and feedback. Staying with the pulse rate example, with electronic biofeedback monitoring equipment, the pulse can be picked up from the fingertip pulse or from EKG sensors. After electronic amplification, the computer converts the pulse to a feedback sound or to a graphics display on a monitor. From the feedback display, you can easily determine the rate of each individual heartbeat, or if you wish, provide an average rate for any specified number of consecutive heartbeats. *The critical feature is that the person whose heart rate is being monitored is the person observing the feedback.* Thus, that person can use that feedback directly to try to alter their heart rate. Depending on the computer software, the feedback display options are almost endless. Ideally the display should be informative and very easy to understand. The goal is to use this feedback to try to raise, lower, or stabilize heart rate. This can be done, of course, only within the natural physiological limits allowed by the body. (See figure 7.1.)

History

It used to be thought that animals and humans possessed little intentional control over such "involuntary" physiological responses as heart rate, blood pressure, stomach motility, skin temperature, sweating, level of brain wave activation, and resting level of muscle tension. Nevertheless, in a variety of animal and human studies in the 1960s, it was demonstrated that, with feedback of the moment-to-moment status of these various functions, both animals and humans could perform more intentional self-regulation than had been previously thought possible.

By the mid-1970s, enthusiastic claims were made about the potential of biofeedback training for treating medical disorders involving disregulation of neurophysiological systems. It has taken another twenty years of research to sort out these claims. Today there is abundant evidence of the value of biofeedback in:

1. Facilitating cognitive and physiological relaxation

2. Promoting general health, healing, and rehabilitation

3. Helping with pain management

Biofeedback's value in headache management has proven to be one of the best substantiated of these claims.

Biofeedback involves attaching sensors to the skin for recording physiologic events such as breathing, muscle tension, heart rate, or sweating. This information is then transferred to a video monitor where it can be used as an aid in learning how to improve self-regulation of these physiologic events.

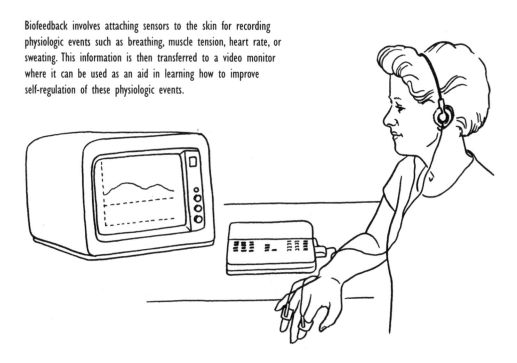

Figure 7.1:   **Biofeedback Monitoring**

Biofeedback does not teach control over functions that can't be learned in some other manner. Its major role seems to be in speeding up the process of learning self-regulation. In cases of low motivation, it can also make self-regulation more interesting. Medical scientists and practitioners have shown a renewed interest in the older techniques of self-regulation because biofeedback, with its scientific roots in experimental psychology, has prompted a widespread interest in the phenomenon of self-regulation.

Common Types (or Modalities) of Biofeedback

The term biofeedback refers to the process of providing physiological feedback. The actual type of feedback is determined by whatever physiological function is of interest and is being monitored and converted to feedback (information) about that function. In addition to *heart rate* there are a number of other commonly used types of biofeedback.

By placing *electromyographic* (EMG) sensors on the skin over a muscle, you can instantly determine the state of muscle tension and whether it is increasing or decreasing. The same can be done with *temperature* sensors on the skin, electrical *skin conductance* to monitor sweat gland activity, or an *electroencephalogram* (EEG) to monitor brain waves. In fact, almost any and every physical function can be converted to an electrical signal that can be converted to feedback.

The potential of biofeedback as a teaching technology goes well beyond teaching relaxation techniques. For example, one of the most effective applications of EMG biofeedback is helping individuals learn exercises to improve control of the muscles involved in bowel and bladder control, and even in sexual functioning. Another example currently under exploration is the use of EEG biofeedback for children with attention deficit disorders; it may be possible to develop brain wave patterns via biofeedback conducive to improved attention and concentration, which may lead to improved learning.

In any particular feedback session, the biofeedback may be from multiple sites on the body, reflecting the functioning of many different systems, or it may from a single system. In general, it's more useful to try to keep it as simple as possible.

Common Medical Uses of Biofeedback

The major medical uses of biofeedback are as follows:

1. Facilitating the learning of general relaxation and pain control techniques by adding biofeedback to the types of self-regulation exercises considered in this workbook. When learning to use focused attention to control physical systems, it's helpful to have a direct measurement gauge for these systems. This is the most common application of biofeedback technology.

2. Aiding muscle rehabilitation of neuromuscular functioning following illness, accidents, and injuries. Patients with spinal cord injuries and stroke patients are common recipients. As with relaxation training, biofeedback serves as a gauge of success for regaining and improving muscle control.

3. Combining 1 and 2 (above) for head and neck pain. That is, combining general relaxation and pain control techniques with muscle rehabilitation of neuromuscular functioning for head and neck pain. Teaching improved bladder and bowel control (as mentioned above) is another example of combining the use of biofeedback to improve both relaxation ability and muscle control.

4. Helping a wide range of special applications related to neuroendocrine regulation, such as control of high blood pressure, orthostatic low blood pressure, gastric motility, respiratory functioning, and impaired peripheral circulation.

Combining Biofeedback with the BMW(I) Formula

Biofeedback informs us of how we're doing as we try to self-regulate. It does nothing to the body; it's merely an elaborate teaching aid. As you follow the (BMW)I formula, it can keep you informed of the rate and depth of your breathing, the tension in your muscles, and the temperature of your hands. This information is typically displayed on a dial or a video monitor.

Learning any skill improves with instant, ongoing feedback. Presumably, you could learn to shoot a basket by only the feel of your jumpshot and by being told after the fact whether you made the basket. But the instant feedback from watching the ball in flight swish through the net is going to be a faster way to learn how to shoot a basket.

If biofeedback were added to the (BMW)I formula followed in this workbook, here's what you would see:

Slow-Deep Breathing

Sensors: Strain gauges are strapped to your chest and abdomen to monitor the rate and depth of your abdominal and chest breathing.

Feedback: A graph might be placed on the feedback video monitor with two electronic tracings representing the two strain gauges moving across the face of the graph. The degree of deflection of the video lines will show the depth and length of each breath. Your instructions are to make the chest tracing become increasing smaller while the abdominal deflection becomes correspondingly larger.

Muscle Relaxation

Sensors: Small, metal EMG (electromyogram) sensors are placed on the muscles of interest—usually the neck, jaw, forehead, and upper back.

Feedback: A similar graph to that described above could be used to represent EMG and ongoing changes in muscle activation from any or all muscles represented by deflections on the lines sweeping across the graph. If your goal is to balance the muscle tension from the two sides of your neck, you could just watch two lines and try to get them to overlap as much as possible. Another possibility for balancing tension from the two sides of your neck might be to display the two EMG outputs as side-by-side bar graphs. Yet another possibility might be to display a video balance beam, similar to a child's teeter-totter, with the balance controlled by the relative level of EMG from each side of your neck.

Hand Warming

Sensors: Temperature sensors taped to your hand(s) or finger(s).

Feedback: Your actual skin temperature, accurate to a .1 degree, might be directly read from a video feedback monitor. Or a simulated thermometer could be displayed on the screen, or a change in color, as in a mood ring. Other popular temperature feedback arrangements include geometric displays that become larger and smaller as your temperature changes.

Other Responses

Obviously there is no direct physiological counterpart of mental imagery that can be monitored. The success of the mental imagery, however, may be reflected in the degree of change seen in the other dimensions.

In addition to the three dimensions of slow-deep breathing, muscle relaxation, and hand warming described above, if you wish to have a fuller picture of autonomic activation, you could also add heart rate and skin conductance monitoring. Other commonly used possibilities include blood pressure and brain waves (EEG). These are some of the most common types of biofeedback, although many other more exotic applications are possible.

Biofeedback for Headaches

Biofeedback-assisted self-regulation training for headaches can proceed just as described above with the monitoring and feedback of breathing, muscle relaxation, and hand temperature. However, most therapists include just EMG muscle and hand temperature feedback, often adding heart rate and skin conductance for a more complete picture of autonomic nervous system (ANS) activation. Respiration is monitored infrequently because technically it can be tedious to get the strain-gauge transducers adjusted, and it's relatively easy for most people to master the slow-deep breathing techniques. Biofeedback probably adds little to the speed of learning slow-deep breath control unless you're having an unusual degree of difficulty with diaphragmatic breathing.

The EMG muscle feedback appears to be the biofeedback modality that's of greatest value for headaches. Of course, the EMG monitoring is useful to identify and try to reduce muscle tension, and to correct patterns of muscle use. As pointed out in chapter 6, headaches related to muscle problems aren't only a consequence of tense muscles, but can also be the result of weak or inefficient and posturally incorrect use of muscles. In that case, EMG feedback may be used both to encourage strengthening of muscles and to help develop an improved pattern of muscle use.

Finally, temperature regulation is used often with migraine and other vascular headaches. As you already know, an irregularity in vasoconstriction followed by vasodilation of the arteries in the scalp seems to be a major feature of many migraine headaches. There is also some evidence that migraine sufferers are prone to experience cold hands as part of a systemic tendency towards vasospastic symptoms. Thus learning how to warm your hands as part of a general relaxation pattern is a key strategy in the long-term control of migraines.

Biofeedback Protocol at the University of Virginia Pain Management Center

The Pain Management Center at the University of Virginia tries to integrate biofeedback into the protocol for teaching self-regulation of headaches in the following manner.

Initial Evaluation

We begin with a review of medical information from referral records and from an interview with the patient.

1. Medical and Psychosocial Screening
   If diagnostic uncertainty remains after the review and interview, further medical exams and laboratory studies are requested. There is a review of past and current medication, and, if necessary, a new medication plan is established. Finally, a brief psychological interview for identifying current life stressors and current and past functioning is conducted.

2. Psychophysiological Baseline and Stress Test
   Patients are comfortably seated in an upright position in a straight-backed chair with their hands placed in their laps. EMG muscle sensors are placed on the forehead and on the trapezius muscles at either side of the base of the neck. Pulse rate, skin conductance, and temperature are monitored from the fingers. These physiological measures are monitored continuously and then reduced to one minute averages for printout.

   The procedure is:

   - Five minutes resting baseline
   - One minute cognitive stressor—mental arithmetic (count backwards from 500 by 7s)
   - Three minutes rest recovery
   - One minute cognitive stressor—H words (say all the words you can think of that start with H)
   - Three minutes rest recovery
   - One minute physical stressor—raise your arms to shoulder level and hold
   - Three minutes rest recovery
   - One minute physical stressor—stand up with your hands at your side
   - Three minutes rest recovery

   The baseline- and stressor-task-monitoring session is brief and easy to conduct. Obviously, it does not reflect real life stressors to any significant degree; nevertheless, it can provide very valuable information. It provides information about resting baselines and adaptation over time. It reveals whether the physical response to minor stressors is normal versus hyper- or hyporeactive. The session also indicates whether the physiological functions rapidly return to resting baseline levels after the stressor is removed. Finally, the bilateral EMG from the neck informs us about degree of muscle symmetry at this critical location.

3. Wrap-Up and Assignments
   The biofeedback therapists review the results of the simple stress test with the patient. In some cases, slow-deep breathing exercises are introduced for beginning home practice. The patient is also given a headache self-monitoring log.

Training Sessions

At four to ten subsequent sessions at weekly intervals, muscular and autonomic functions are monitored with the patient seated in a semirecumbent position in which the body is fully supported by the chair.

1. Review of Progress
   Progress and/or problems indicated by the logs are noted and discussed with the therapist. The patient is asked to continue with the self-monitoring logs and to return them at each appointment.

2. Self-Regulation Instruction
   The therapists discuss the Scan, Focus, (BMW)I strategies and the training proceeds as described in chapters 4 and 5. Depending on the indications from the initial evaluation session, extra time may be spent on bilateral EMG from the neck to try to reduce tension in this critical area, and to improve the bilateral symmetry of muscle functioning.

   During later sessions, the EMG biofeedback may continue while the patient sits upright or stands in an effort to generalize muscle control to areas with increased postural demands. Some patients also receive exercise or physical therapy to try to improve muscle tone and functioning. Likewise, some receive extra training in hand warming with biofeedback where cold hands and feet appear to be a dominant feature.

3. Supportive Counseling
   Counseling that focuses on identifying stressors and/or personal perceptions is added as necessary.

Completion of Training

The average number of sessions is four to ten, although the range is considerable. Some people already are quite skilled at self-regulation from the start, and need to be reminded only how to make better systematic use of that skill for dealing with their headaches. Others take longer before developing the confidence that they can use their skill to modify and even prevent headaches. Some patients return for an occasional follow-up booster session every month or two for several months.

It is extremely important to keep up the (BMW)I home practice. You must also develop the minimum application along with the instinctive reflex to scan for increases in tension and use it as a cue to "let go" (i.e., self-regulate) wherever you are.

One advantage of learning (BMW)I skills without biofeedback is that it becomes obvious that this is something you are doing yourself and can use anywhere. Obviously, you can't carry biofeedback equipment with you everywhere you go. You must develop confidence that whatever you can accomplish with biofeedback, in time and with practice, you can also do without it. If you're going to permanently alter a persistent pattern of chronic headaches long after your formal training is completed, you must continue Scan, Focus, and follow with the (BMW)I maximum and minimum applications until they become a way of life.

Summary

For any headache control technique that requires a person to learn new skills and to practice those skills, the process *must engage the interest, motivation, and effort of the individual*. For that reason biofeedback can be a powerful teaching tool. If learning to follow the (BMW)I formula of self-regulation seems just too abstract or difficult, you might do better at learning self-regulation with biofeedback.

Key Word Summary

To ensure that you have thoroughly mastered the material in this chapter, write the definition of each term below in your own words.

Biofeedback: _____

_____

_____

Modalities: _____

_____

_____

Baseline: _____

_____

_____

Stress test: _____

_____

_____

Recovery: _____

_____

_____

Further Readings:

Nigl, A. J. 1984. *Biofeedback and Behavioral Strategies in Pain Treatment.* Jamaica, NY: Spectrum Publications.

Olton, D. S. and A. R. Noonberg. 1980. *Biofeedback: Clinical Applications in Behavioral Medicine.* Englewood Cliffs, NJ: Prentice-Hall.

Schwartz, Mark S. 1995. *Biofeedback: A Practitioner's Guide.* 2nd ed. New York: Guilford Publications.

Chapter 8

Drug Treatment for Headaches

Donald C. Manning, M.D., Ph.D.

▲ Medications for nausea and vomiting

▲ Medications for migraine treatment

▲ Medications for migraine prevention

▲ Medications for tension-type headache

▲ Preventive therapy for cluster headaches

Traditionally, headaches have been attributed to blood vessel diameter or muscle tension, as well as to inflammation mechanisms. In this chapter, I have kept to this mechanistic scheme, but you should be aware that newer studies suggest that headaches all share certain characteristics. This newer way of approaching headaches allows for the same types of drugs to treat several different types of headache.

Traditional teaching attributes migraine aura to a diffuse constriction of blood vessels outside the brain followed by dilation during the headache's painful phase. Dilation causes increased activity in the nerves surrounding the blood vessels, which can lead to inflammation around the vessels. Migraine is the classic vascular headache, and its treatment is centered on relieving the dilation with vasoconstrictive agents and treating the pain with analgesics and anti-inflammatory agents.

Muscular tension in the neck and head is often associated with anxiety and depression. Thus, both emotional strain and muscle tension may jointly lead to the head and neck pain of chronic tension headaches. Chronic tension headaches are treated by addressing the stress, anxiety, and depression partly with antidepressants and muscle relaxants with vasoconstrictive agents.

In this chapter, medications for each as well as primary type of headache will be divided into

- Abortive treatments for attempting to control a headache in progress
- Drugs for the prevention of headache onset

This distinction is extremely important because some of the drugs used to relieve an acute headache may actually *cause* headache if used for its prophylaxis (cure and/or prevention). Migraine receives the most attention here because most problematic headaches either are migraines or have features of migraines, combined with other types of headache symptoms.

Note that most drugs are listed by their chemical name(s) followed by brand name(s) in parentheses, where appropriate.

Treatment of Nausea and Vomiting

Serious headaches are often accompanied by nausea and vomiting. Unless the nausea, vomiting, and sound and light sensitivity associated with the headache can be reduced, treating the headache pain may be very difficult.

Nausea-Suppressing Drugs

The following drugs are used to combat nausea.

Anticholinergics

The most commonly used anticholinergic substance for treating nausea is *trimethobenzamide* (Tigan). Anticholinergic drugs usually have symptoms with very noticeable side effects including confusion in older people, alteration in intestinal motility, urinary retention, and dry mouth.

Antidopaminergics

These highly tranquilizing drugs include *chlorpromazine* (Thorazine), *prochlorperazine* (Compazine), and *thiethylperazine* (Torecan). Serious side effects with long-term use are the risk of Parkinsonian-like tremor and oversedation.

Antihistamines

Diphenhydramine (Benadryl), *hydroxyzine* (Vistaril), and *promethazine* (Phenergan) are the best known of these drugs. Side effects include drowsiness, anxiety, dizziness, and dry mouth.

Gastrokinetic (Antivomiting) Agents

Metoclopramide (Reglan) is the most frequently used gastrokinetic agent. It stimulates stomach and intestinal motility to move stomach contents onward and thus reduce nausea. It can also improve the absorption of medications taken orally during a migraine attack. Its major side effect is Parkinsonian-like muscle tremors. It should not be taken if you're pregnant, have low blood pressure, have a history of seizures, or if you're taking neuroleptic (tranquilizing) drugs.

Migraine Headaches

Migraine headaches are common and attacks occur episodically and usually last for only a few hours. Some patients with migraine have visual and skin sensations of short duration before the headache starts. These early sensations are called "aura" symptoms. Many migraine sufferers do not have aura symptoms and have just the abrupt onset of a headache. Migraine is often treated with drugs when the patient cannot function because of the intense pain.

Acute Abortive Treatment of Migraine

Think of migraine headaches as an episodic widening or dilation of the blood vessels outside the brain, and it becomes easy to see why the drugs that constrict blood vessels can give relief from the headache pain.

Several considerations are relevant to selecting a drug for migraine treatment. You must be sure that the attack *is* a migraine because some of the therapies directed toward blood vessels will not be effective in other headache types and can lead to overuse and a rebound headache. Is the attack mild or severe? Sometimes, attacks can vary in intensity. Mild attacks may be treated with aspirin, while the more potent and side-effect laden drugs can be reserved for severe attacks, minimizing overuse. Your doctor will need to consider any other medical conditions that you may have when helping you to select the best drug. Significant conditions include heart disease, pregnancy, and high blood pressure. The route of administration of the drug can be important if severe nausea and vomiting are involved. When you can't take oral medications, your doctor may prescribe injectable medications or rectal suppositories to help you through the worst attack.

Your choice of a drug to abort your headache also depends upon its intensity and how long it lasts. If your headache occurs during the day and you can take a medication right away, then oral analgesics or vasoconstrictive agents are used. Oral agents will be effective early in the headache before the stomach and intestinal effects of your headache prevent absorption of the drug. If you wake up with a full-blown headache, it's best to start with a medication to increase stomach and bowel motility fifteen minutes before taking the analgesic. This strategy works best to provide good absorption of the drug and a better effect. If the analgesics are taken too soon, then the vasoconstrictor or analgesic medications will be taken too often and lead to increased frequency of headaches. Analgesics have increased efficacy when combined with gastrokinetic agents such as Reglan. These agents relieve your nausea and improve the absorption of oral medications.

Nonnarcotic Analgesics

Analgesics provide immediate relief to help stop the pain of migraine once it has started. These agents tend to act fast, but they last only a short period (three to six hours). If your headaches are frequent or prolonged, you may be tempted to overuse these agents. Overuse can lead to a medication dependency such that when the dose wears off you'll have a rebound headache and you'll need more medication and will get shorter periods of relief. It's therefore important that you limit the amount and dosage of these drugs. If the headache is prolonged, you should see your doctor or use more appropriate therapy. You may be surprised to learn that this rebound problem can occur even with the most common analgesics, such as acetaminophen and aspirin. Keeping that in mind, the following medications can be very effective if used for a limited period of time.

Acetaminophen (Tylenol). Acetaminophen acts within the central nervous system to relieve pain. It has a minimum number of side effects, but it must not be taken with alcohol or in total doses over 4000 milligrams (mgs) a day. This is the drug of choice for people with ulcers or stomach irritation.

Aspirin has demonstrated effectiveness against migraine and compares favorably to acetaminophen. The efficacy approaches 42 percent for improvement and relief of migraine. The most common side effects with heavy use are stomach irritation, abnormal bleeding, ringing in the ears, and vertigo.

Nonsteroidal anti-inflammatory agents. Ibuprofen (Motrin, Advil), *naproxen* (Naprosyn), *naproxen sodium* (Anaprox), *mefenamic acid* (Ponstel), and *Indomethacin* (Indocin). These drugs inhibit the production of inflammatory chemicals and relieve both pain and inflammation. They have their effect both in the periphery and within the central nervous system. In particular, Indocin is a potent analgesic, vasoconstrictor and inhibitor of neurogenic inflammation. Many patients can't tolerate these agents due to their ability to cause stomach irritation, kidney damage, and blood clotting problems. In general, however, these drugs are safe to use over short periods of time and can be very effective in treating mild headaches.

Narcotic Analgesics: Opioids

Despite the apparent logic in using opiate medications for pain, there's very little evidence for their use in chronic (long-term) therapy for headache. The most appropriate use of opiates is for the short-term treatment of acute, high-intensity headache. This treatment should take place preferably in a hospital where dosing and effectiveness can be monitored. The opioid drugs are very effective for acute pain relief. One of the most common side effects is nausea, which usually makes opioids difficult to take for migraine sufferers. Most of the common opioids don't last for very long, and they can lead to dependence and rebound headache. Many studies have indicated that opioids aren't good agents for long-term treatment of headache because patients develop a tolerance to the drug and they don't directly address the headache mechanisms.

Codeine is the weakest but most commonly used opioid for headaches. It's administered most often with acetaminophen or aspirin. Occasionally, it's combined with caffeine. Codeine must be converted to morphine within the body, but up to 7 percent of patients can't perform this conversion and, therefore, would get very little analgesic relief from codeine. For those patients who can convert codeine, it's approximately 50 percent effective for headache relief.

Meperidine (Demerol) is often given by injection in the ER for the treatment of an acute migraine attack. Typically, its effects last two to three hours, which can lead to multiple doses if the headache is prolonged. The oral form of meperidine isn't well absorbed by the intestine and isn't very useful for headache therapy. Chronic use of meperidine, especially in those with impaired kidney function, can lead to the buildup of a toxic by-product and lead to seizures.

Butorphanol (Stadol) has been marketed as an effective treatment for aborting a migraine episode. It's delivered intranasally (through the nasal structure), thereby effecting a faster delivery of the drug. Butorphanol doesn't have the same side effects as morphine or codeine, such as respiratory depression and constipation, but it does have the potential for overuse and precipitation of a rebound headache. (Stadol's potential for physical dependency and addiction have been reported with increasing frequency.) Problems have been reported with the intranasal sprayer; sometimes it delivers the proper dose of medication but frequently it malfunctions if it isn't primed properly. Your doctor or pharmacist can assist you in the proper use of this device.

Hydrocodone (Vicoden, Lorcet) is often used for *moderately* severe acute pain, while *morphine* and *oxycodone* (Perocet) are used for more *severe* acute pain. Morphine is readily available in an injectable form and can be used for emergency treatment of headache. In general, however, these drugs shouldn't be used routinely to treat headaches because of the significant risks listed earlier. Chronic use of potent opioids is most appropriate for *constant* pain. *Episodic* pain such as headache usually leads to escalating opioid dosage because these drugs are ineffective under such conditions.

Vasoconstrictive Agents

Vasoconstrictors that mimic the sympathetic nervous system actions include:

Isometheptene. This agent will reduce the size of blood vessels within the scalp to abort a headache. It's used most commonly in combination with a mild sedative (dichloralphenazone) and an analgesic (acetaminophen), such as in the preparation of Midrin. Combination agents such as Midrin are appropriate when aspirin or other nonsteroidal, anti-inflammatory agents can't be used because of ulcer or asthma. Too frequent use can lead to dependence and rebound headache. Side effects include dizziness, sedation, and circulatory disturbances. Contraindications include glaucoma, use of monoamine oxidase inhibitors (MAOI) within two weeks, porphyria, severe renal disease, hypertension, heart disease, and liver disease.

Serotonergic Vasoconstrictors

These agents both constrict the blood vessels outside the brain and reduce the inflammation that can occur around the blood vessels during a headache that leads to pain. Due to the potency of their blood vessel–contracting properties, these agents aren't to be used if you have hypertension or coronary heart disease, because of the risk of stroke or heart attack.

Ergot alkaloids. This group of drugs has been used for many years and is available in several forms, including oral, subcutaneous (under the skin), and rectal and sublingual (under the tongue). Efficacy for headache resolution depends upon the route of administration. Ergots are effective within the first one to two hours in 90 percent of patients when given intravenously or subcutaneously, 80 percent effective by the rectal route, and 50 percent effective orally. The lower efficacy in the oral route is partly due to the decreased stomach and intestinal motility seen with headache and also due to the ergot itself.

Ergotamine tartrate (Ergomar, Wigrettes, Wigraine, and Ergostat). This group of drugs is the oldest and most effective form of ergot but it also has the most side effects. Dihydroergotamine (DHE-45) is the only intravenous form available and although it has fewer side effects, it is not as effective as ergotamine. A combination of ergotamine and caffeine is marketed as Cafergot, available both as a tablet and a suppository. The addition of caffeine helps your body to absorb the ergot drug. Bellergal is a combination drug containing ergotamine tartrate, belladonna, and barbiturate. A sustained-release preparation is called Bellergal-S. Some patients have found this agent useful, but like all ergots, it can be used only for short periods to prevent dependence.

There are considerable problems with the use of ergotamine. Because of the significant danger in chronic dosing with this drug, it is reserved for short-term pain prevention only. Ergotamine tartrate preparations should not be used more than two days per week. If they're used for prolonged periods, rebound headaches can occur and peripheral blood vessels can become abnormally constricted and lead to leg cramps, abdominal cramps, and, in severe cases, gangrene in the legs. Other reported side effects include nausea/vomiting, tingling in the hands and feet, swollen fingers, diarrhea, tremor, and fainting. Contraindications for ergotamine use include cardiovascular disease (coronary heart disease, heart rhythm disturbances, uncontrolled hypertension), pregnancy, breast feeding, liver or kidney disease, severe infection, and the use of erythromycin. Use ergotamine with caution if you're taking sumatriptan, methysergide, or beta blockers. Safety is also unclear when ergotamine is used during a migraine attack with aura.

Sumatriptan (Imitrex). This is one of the newest agents on the market to treat migraine. It most likely has its analgesic effect by constricting blood vessels. It's effective against nausea, vomiting, and light and sound sensitivity. It can be given during both the aura or warning period, or late in the attack, without a change in efficacy. The most effective form is an autoinjector device to deliver the medication under the skin. An oral form is available, but it is not as effective against migraine symptoms. Once taken, sumatriptan can be effective quickly, but in some people the relief can be delayed for up to two hours. If the first dose is ineffective, a second dose will be of little use. If the first dose is effective but the headache returns, another dose can be taken to help prevent the return of the headache. It's important to understand that the second dose doesn't increase the relief, it just helps prevent the return of the headache. If you find that you're taking sumatriptan every day for several days, then the headache is probably not a migraine, but possibly a chronic tension headache or a drug-maintained headache (rebound).

Like other drugs that constrict blood vessels, sumatriptan shouldn't be used if you have a history of heart attack or angina, as it can precipitate another heart attack. It's common, however, for patients taking sumatriptan by injection to feel a heaviness in their chest, tingling, flushed and burning sensations in various body regions, and possibly some pain at the site of the injection.

Summary: Abortive Treatment of Migraine

The standard approach to acute migraine treatment depends on the time of onset and how early in the course you can take the medication. If your headache occurs during the day, then the slower acting but more convenient and less toxic agents can be used if your headache is mild. You can start with an antinausea medication such as Reglan and follow it with aspirin, ibuprofen, or acetaminophen. If your headache is severe, then Midrin, Naprosyn, Indomethacin, or sumatriptan (oral form) can be taken. On the other hand, if your headache is present when you wake up, or if it occurs during the night, more potent agents will need to be used. A full-intensity headache usually requires injectable or rectal therapy, because the stomach and intestine have already been affected. The agents of choice are then an Indocin suppository, sumatriptan injection, Cafergot suppository, or dihydroergotamine subcutaneously or intramuscularly. Opioids can be useful only for the occasional severe headache.

Medications for the Prevention of Migraine

Preventive therapy may be considered if:

- Your migraine attacks are more frequent than one or two per month

- Your migraines impair your normal activities

- Your migraines cause severe emotional trauma

- Abortive therapies don't work, or cause serious side effects

When choosing a preventive therapy regimen, your doctor will take several factors into consideration. It's usually wise to keep a headache diary for at least one month to help determine the frequency of your headaches, their predictability, and associated symptoms. These will be taken into consideration in addition to any other medical problems that you may have, such as heart disease, asthma, stomach ulcers, or high blood pressure.

Short-Term Prevention

Drug therapy for the prevention of migraine can be carried out over a short period, or long term. The choice of drug therapy depends upon when and how frequently your migraines occur. When your headaches are less frequent but predictable, the ergot drugs such as Bellergal-S can be taken at bedtime, for one to two days before the expected headache. Methysergide can be used for short-term prevention as long as the dosing periods are short, and fibrosis (scarring) can be avoided. Nonsteroidal anti-inflammatory agents, such as Naproxen, can be used for short-term prevention, as well. Short-term use of these agents will not usually produce stomach irritation.

Menstrual migraines are an episodic, infrequent, but predictable headache and occur commonly around the start of the menstrual period. Most commonly, nonsteroidal drugs such as Naproxen and mefenamic acid (Ponstel) are used for menstrual migraine–headache prevention. The dosing begins three days before the menses and continues until spotting stops. Ergotamine is also commonly used for this short period before the menstrual flow starts.

Long-Term Prevention

Methysergide. In the past, methysergide (Sansert) had been the standard drug for migraine prevention with 50 to 65 percent efficacy. The way methysergide works isn't known, but it may involve interfering with serotonin to prevent both vasodilatation and vasoconstriction. Serious side effects, however, limit its use today. The most common side effects are muscle aching, abdominal pain and discomfort, hallucinations, and a sense of swelling around the face or throat. Often these disappear with continued dosing. Chronic dosing, however, can also be a problem. Methysergide should not be taken for more than five to six months without a break of one to two months. Taking this drug for longer periods can lead to fibrosis in the abdomen, lungs, and heart valves, which isn't always reversible. Methysergide should not be used if you have peripheral vascular disease or hypertension, if you are pregnant, or if you have intestinal pain or disease.

Beta-receptor Blockers. Currently the first choice for long-term prevention is often the beta blockers, such as *propranolol* (Inderal and Inderal LA) or *timolol* (Blocadren). Only propranolol and timolol are approved for migraine therapy, although several other beta-receptor blockers appear to have some effect on preventing headaches. These include *atenolol* (Tenormin), *metoprolol* (Lopressor), and *nadolol* (Corgard). The primary use of beta blockers is to reduce the sympathetic nervous system actions, thus they tend to reduce blood pressure and heart rate activation. Be careful if you are asthmatic, because some beta blockers can precipitate an asthma attack. The preferred beta blockers for asthmatics are timolol, atenolol, and metoprolol, because of their ability to selectively affect blood vessels and the heart without much effect on the lungs. Unfortunately, the less selective drugs (e.g., Tenormin, Lopressor, Corgard) have been shown to be the most effective for prevention of migraines.

Antidepressants. The second choice for long-term prevention is the tricyclic antidepressants, such as *amitriptyline* (Elavil). The tricyclic class of antidepressant has several uses in addition to the treatment of depression. These antidepressants have been used to treat a wide variety of pain conditions including headache. They are best suited for chronic therapy, as the analgesic effect is often delayed and it can take days or even weeks to reach the therapeutic dose. The most effective antidepressant and the best studied in this regard is amitriptyline (Elavil). Amitriptyline is especially indicated for migraines if you have asthma, or are having problems with sleep. Amitriptyline is long acting and therefore is taken once a day, usually at night. It's also useful for the prophylaxis of migraine headache. Other drugs in this same class don't seem to have as good an effect on treating or preventing headaches. Side effects include dry mouth, weight gain, skin reactions, nausea, constipation, and urinary retention. You should not use these agents if you're pregnant, have problems with urinary retention, have heart disease, seizures, or are taking monoamine oxidase inhibitors. Use antidepressants with caution if you have glaucoma, or liver, kidney, or thyroid disease.

Fluvoxamine (Luvox) is a new antidepressant that acts on serotonin. It has fewer side effects than most antidepressants and can lead to weight loss. Side effects can include nausea, flu-like symptoms, and jitteriness.

Monoamine oxidase (MAOI) inhibitors are yet another class of antidepressant agents that have been used to treat headaches. The most common agents are *phenelzine* (Nardil) and *isocarboxazid* (Marplan). These agents have to be carefully monitored by a physician, and you should avoid eating foods containing *tyramine*, such as aged cheese and red wine. Also, you should avoid taking MAOI inhibitors with other drugs, such as *meperidine* (Demerol), and decongestants, such as Contact, Dristan, Sinutabs, or decongestant nose drops.

Other MAOI inhibitors include verapamil, valproate, aspirin, clonidine, and cyproheptadine.

Calcium Entry Blockers. *Verapamil* (Isoptin) and *nifedipine* (Procardia) are agents that can reduce or prevent several possible migraine mechanisms. They can both inhibit the release of chemical mediators of inflammation, and influence blood vessel size to reduce the constriction and the active dilation. The full benefit may be delayed until three to four weeks after starting the medication. Verapamil should not be used with certain types of congestive heart failure or if you have a condition where your heartbeat is irregular. Side effects can include low blood pressure, heart rhythm disturbances, swelling, constipation, worsening of headaches, depression, and nausea. There may be a transient increase in your headaches when you first start taking the drug.

Miscellaneous Medications. *Cyproheptadine* (Periactin), a serotonin receptor–activating drug, has had only limited success in preventing migraine attacks in adults, but its safety makes it the drug of choice for children with migraine. Significant side effects include dry mouth, drowsiness, appetite stimulation, and weight gain.

Clonidine (Catapres) isn't FDA-approved for migraine but it has proven effective for other pain states. Clonidine can inhibit the sympathetic nervous system and the brain to influence blood vessels and give pain relief. Most uses of clonidine are limited by the prominent side effects of drowsiness, dry mouth, constipation, ejaculation difficulties, and dizziness. Dangerous interactions can occur when taken with antidepressants. You should not stop taking clonidine abruptly because it can cause severe high blood pressure during withdrawal. You should taper the dose over two to four days under your physician's supervision.

Valproate (Depakote, Valproex) is an antiseizure drug that is now available in a long-acting formulation. Consistent use of valproate has been successful in preventing migraines, cluster, and chronic daily headaches. Significant side effects include nausea, drowsiness, bleeding easily, hair loss, and liver toxicity. Excessive sedation can occur if you take valproate with tricyclic antidepressants, barbiturates, or Valium-like compounds.

Finally, the anti-inflammatory medications *aspirin* and *naproxen sodium* (Anaprox) occasionally can play a role in preventing migraines.

Conclusion

Most preventive therapy must be continued for at least six months, then the dose can be decreased very slowly to prevent rebound headache during the withdrawal. You may end up at a lower dose for an extended period of time without a recurrence of headaches. Occasionally the medication can be eliminated altogether. You should discuss these options and adjust the dose only in collaboration with your doctor. Most medications used to prevent migraines are effective between 50 to 60 percent of the time. Less effective therapies in the 30 to 40 percent range are ergotamine, aspirin, and clonidine.

Tension-Type Headache

The so-called "muscular tension" headaches aren't due entirely to muscle contraction. Most studies of muscle-relaxant drugs for treatment of tension headaches have had poor results. For some people, however, there does appear to be some benefit from *cyclobenzaprine* (Flexeril) and *meprobamate* (Soma), but no information is available on the long-term effects. There is no established benefit from the benzodiazepines (Valium, Xanax) or other tranquilizing agents. Because there is so much overlap between the symptoms of tension-type headache and migraine, many of the medications discussed in the migraine section will reappear here. If you have any coexisting depression, it should be treated regardless of whether drugs improve your headaches. Coping skills for dealing with your headaches can then be optimized when your depression is under control.

Acute Treatment of Tension Headaches

Acute drug therapy for a headache in progress is directed at the most prominent symptom. The muscular pain is treated with familiar analgesics such as aspirin, acetaminophen, and ibuprofen, and the migraine symptoms are treated with vasoconstrictive agents, such as ergotamines or sumatriptan. The choice of drug is limited mostly by the intended length of time of the therapy. Opiates, barbiturates, and caffeine can be effective for the acute attack but are inappropriate for long-term use.

The combination medications are especially useful here. Many of the combination agents contain *butalbital*, which is a weak barbiturate used as a sedative. Several commonly used combination agents and their chemical components are as follows:

- Aspirin, caffeine, and butalbital (Fiorinal)

- Acetaminophen, caffeine, and butalbital (Fioricet, Esgic)

- Aspirin, caffeine, butalbital, and codeine (Fiorinol with codeine)

- Acetaminophen, isometheptene, and dichloralphenazone (Midrin)

- Butalbital and acetaminophen (Phreniline)

Using a combination of medications may also lower the risk of side effects because then lower doses of each medication can be used. The combinations often include an analgesic, a sedative, and a vasoconstrictor. This combination treats not only the perception of pain but also the reaction to pain, which may contribute to the muscular spasms.

Preventive Therapy

Quick relief for the occasional tension-type headache is much easier to accomplish than is prevention of severe chronic headaches. Tension headaches can become quite chronic, therefore the prevention strategies should avoid dependence-producing agents. The tricyclic antidepressants are the preventive therapy of choice for long-term use because of the high incidence of depression among headache patients, as well as their effects on regulating serotonin. Tricyclic antidepressants are also useful for regulating your sleep patterns. Several drugs that should not be used to prevent chronic, tension-type headaches include opiates, ergotamine, barbiturates, tranquilizers, and caffeine.

Chronic tension headaches tend to occur in cyclical fashion. You should discuss plans for eventually discontinuing the medication once your current episode has been relieved. In the usual situation, 80 percent improvement should be maintained for three to four months, then the medication should be tapered. Tapering should be gradual, with 20 to 25 percent decrease every two to three days to avoid a rebound headache. If your headache returns or, the dose should be restarted, and the tapering should be delayed.

Cluster Headache

Cluster headaches can be severe and can challenge your drug therapy. They are more common in men, and can occur more frequently during changes in seasons. One or more attacks can occur each day and the pattern can continue for several weeks. Some researchers believe that changes in people's schedules and sleep-wake cycles may be responsible for the initiation of these headaches. Therapy, therefore, is aimed not only at treating and preventing your headaches, but is also aimed at regulating your sleep cycles. You can regulate your daily habits by using tricyclic antidepressants to improve your sleep and by eliminating alcohol, caffeine, and tobacco.

Acute Treatment

Inhaling pure *oxygen* is the standard abortive treatment for cluster headaches. Interestingly, using oxygen isn't effective until the headache has reached its peak severity, and has little effect on the reoccurrence of the headache.

Sumatriptan or ergotamine preparations can be given by injection once your headache has developed. The opiates are avoided usually because using them daily can lead to an unwanted physical dependence.

Preventive Therapy

Prednisone, a corticosteroid medication, is perhaps the most useful and effective drug for fast, preventive control of cluster headaches. There are many strategies for the use of prednisone, but a typical approach is one that uses a three-week course followed by a five-day taper of the dose. Reducing a steroid dose can be problematic because a rebound headache can occur. Steroid prevention therapy is used to ensure headache prevention for people who are traveling, or are away from medical care, and for people who are withdrawing from other headache therapies. The risk from this short-term use of steroids is small, but it is not recommended for people with diabetes or other endocrine diseases.

Lithium carbonate, a drug normally used to control severe mood swings, is effective for preventing cluster headaches in more than 60 percent of sufferers. Good effect can often be accomplished with a lower dose than that used to treat depression. Long-term use is not recommended and frequent "drug holidays," where the medication is withdrawn, may be necessary. Side effects are common and include nausea, vomiting, diarrhea, tremor, blurred vision, and, especially in the summer, dehydration. Lithium carbonate should not be taken in combination with nonsteroidal analgesics to prevent kidney injury.

Ergotamine drugs can be used for short periods of time. Use them carefully until your headaches have stopped, but don't use them for more than four weeks. *Verapamil* can also be effective for prevention, but the doses tend to be higher than those used for hypertension, and the effect can be delayed for several weeks.

Complications of Analgesic Drug Use

No discussion of medications for headaches is complete without restating the risks and complications associated with drug treatment. This is why it's so important that you and your doctor have a carefully worked out plan and don't become careless in your use of these medications. The difficulties inherent in drug management are also a reason why the self-regulation techniques described in this workbook are so important. Less medication is often required if you're proficient in the use of these self-regulation techniques.

Drug Overuse and Rebound Headaches

Drug therapy for headaches is probably the most common treatment offered, even though medications can have harmful effects. Drugs can be used to prevent headaches and to stop headache attacks after they've started, but the use of medications can also maintain a headache during periods of withdrawal from the medication. Short-acting immediate relief agents can lead to rebound headaches when used too frequently or for too long a time. Drug dependence can occur with acetaminophen just as it can occur with opiates. There are several criteria that indicate drug overuse:

1. Taking more than 100 aspirin or aspirin compounds per month

2. Using ergot or 10 mg of ergotamine tartrate daily

3. Taking more than 20 tablets of codeine per week

4. Taking more than 20 capsules of Darvon per week

5. Taking barbiturates, sedatives, or mixed compounds containing these substances consistently

Excessive use of acute pain-relieving drugs is one of the most common factors in converting an episodic headache pattern into a chronic daily headache. In general, chronic pain conditions shouldn't be treated the same as acute pain conditions. The use of immediate-relief drugs can lead to a dependence upon these agents, leading to rebound pain during the period of low drug concentration. This, in turn, leads to an increased use of the drugs, and the cycle becomes more severe. The most commonly abused or overused drugs are acetaminophen and aspirin, often in combination with caffeine and/or a barbiturate. The treatment for this condition is the withdrawal of all analgesic. This represents a difficult and often monumental task for individuals and their physicians. This can be accomplished in the outpatient setting, but occasionally hospitalization is required. Upwards of 50 percent or more of people withdrawn from chronic medication have no need to return to medication because their rebound pain pattern is relieved. Even if the pain isn't relieved, it is rarely worse when you are off the medication. If the medication taper is difficult for someone, longer-acting analgesics, especially nonsteroidal anti-inflammatory agents, can be substituted for the shorter-acting acute pain agents.

Barbiturate- and ergotamine-dependence often require hospitalization for specialized withdrawal programs. Ergotism precipitated by increasing daily usage of ergotamine is manifested by severe constriction of blood vessels in the legs, can lead to loss of blood flow, and, in the most severe cases, gangrene. Ergotism therefore should be treated quickly and often involves abrupt cessation of the drug and substitution with intravenous *dihydroergotamine* to control headaches. In other withdrawal regimens, tricyclic antidepressants are slowly increased in dosage to control the headaches. If barbiturates have been part of the analgesic regimen, the withdrawal should be gradual and under a physician's guidance. Abrupt withdrawal from barbiturates can lead to seizures, which can be delayed in onset for several weeks.

During the withdrawal period from medication you will need to be supported emotionally and psychologically to undergo the difficult time ahead. If anxiety or depression has contributed to the medication overuse, then behavioral techniques may allow a less stressful withdrawal. Under a physician's care and with great regulation, the medication that was overused can be restarted if it's the only one to relieve pain, but the dosing must be controlled.

Toxicity of Analgesics

Methysergide can lead to retroperitoneal fibrosis (scar tissue formation within the abdominal cavity and chest), which can entrap nerves and internal organs in fibrous scar. The symptoms of retroperitoneal fibrosis where the ureters are constricted are lower back pain, leg pain, and urinary difficulty. If even a suspicion of this condition is raised, the drug should be discontinued immediately.

In addition to the development of dependence, acetaminophen, aspirin, and nonsteroidal compounds can have toxic effects on body organs if taken too often or for too long a period of time. Thus, remember that even over-the-counter medications must be used wisely.

Conclusion

Usually, the majority of acute headaches can be controlled by medications. The concerns regarding toxicity and overuse outlined above apply to most medications when used for extended periods of time. On the positive side, as you can see from this chapter, your physician does have a wide range of medication options. If used carefully, a strategy can be developed for dealing with both acute headache pain and for prophylaxis of future headaches. It's important to remember that if your headache is severe, prolonged, or new, you should seek the advice of a physician sooner rather than later. Your doctor is best suited to determine if the headache is a sign of a more worrisome disease, and to develop a plan for the careful use of medications. Finally, keep in mind that research (Matthew, 1981) has demonstrated that for severe headache problems, medications used in combination with self-regulation training produce better results than either therapy used alone.

Further Reading

Spierings, E. L. H., ed. 1996. *Management of Migraine.* Boston: Butterworth-Heinemann.

Diamond S. and D. J. Dalessio, eds. 1992. *The Practicing Physician's Approach to Headache.* 5th ed. Baltimore: Williams & Wilkins.

Tollison, C. D., J. R. Satterthwaite, and J. W. Tollison, eds. 1994. *Handbook of Pain Management.* 2nd ed. Baltimore: Williams & Wilkins.

Olesen, J., P. TfeltHansen, and K. M. A. Welch, eds. 1993. *The Headache.* New York: Raven Press.

CHAPTER 9

Clearing Your Mind: Changing Your Life

▲ Review of stress headache model

▲ Think about stressors

▲ Clarify your stressors, personal perceptions, and personality

▲ Counseling for your headaches

The purpose of this chapter is to look at the actual sources of your stress. Some behavioral suggestions for tackling stressors and personal perceptions of stress are given, and the contributions of counseling are described.

Review of Stress Headache Model

Let's return for a moment to the basic model, relating stress reactions to life stressors, as presented in chapter 1. This model is identical to the one presented in chapter 1, but now let's examine the modifiers of your reactions to life's stressors—*personal perceptions* and *coping resources*. Although most of this workbook is about self-regulation as a coping skill, this chapter focuses on the second element of coping resources—the capacity to change or control the sources of life stress. (See figure 9.1.)

Within this model, *stressors* are defined as the pressures exerted by those people or events around us that challenge our ability to cope.

Personal perception is defined as how you uniquely perceive the stressors in your life, based on your current and past life experience. Differences in personal

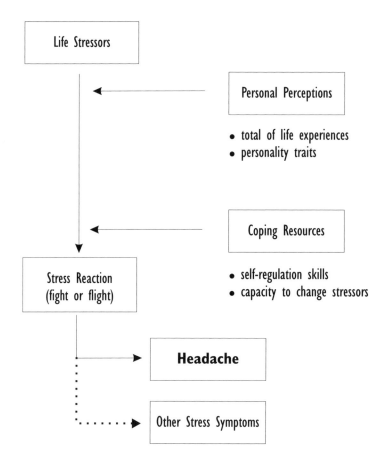

Figure 9.1:   Basic Stress Headache Model

perception can explain why a headache that's just a nuisance for one person can set off feelings of depression in a second person, or great anxiety in a third. Also, personality traits such as perfectionism, compulsiveness, and impatience may contribute to physiological activation and feelings of stress.

Coping resources are considered to be your capacity to control the sources of stress (i.e., the stressors) in your life, as well as your ability to self-regulate your cognitive and physiological reactions to stressors.

Stress reactivity is defined as the impact of stressors on your mind and body. Your stress reactivity, of which headaches can be one symptom, is a result of both the stressors you face, and your genetic or acquired biological diathesis (vulnerability). Other factors influencing the severity of stress reactivity are personal perceptions of stressors and personal coping resources.

Think About Stressors

While you're taking the time to learn self-regulation skills to protect yourself from the cognitive and physiological impact of stressors, it's also a good time to take an inventory of the sources of stress in your life. Is there anything you can do about reducing or eliminating some of those stressors?

For many of you there will be those stressors you can't change, or even stressors you might not want to change—a pregnancy, a new job, even a vacation—all may be enjoyable but nevertheless stressful. There may also, however, be circumstances that you need to identify and modify if you are to ever reduce the constant headache-producing pressures under which you live. You may be able to tackle these stressors on your own, but you should also consider whether professional counseling is needed.

Clarifying Stressors, Personal Perceptions, and Personality

Stressors and personal perceptions that are relevant to your headaches can include

1. The direct consequences of the headaches themselves

2. The many other stressful circumstances in your daily life

3. Personal perceptions and personality traits that may be emotionally linked with headaches

Consequences of Headaches

Headaches can produce misery that goes beyond the actual physical pain sensations. Because of chronic headaches you may begin to feel guilty about not being dependable and not meeting the expectations of others. Compromised job performance may be placing your financial livelihood and career in jeopardy. Keeping up social functions can become so difficult that your friends, spouse, or children may begin to complain. In time, your self-confidence may become badly shaken. Your sleep may be disturbed, appetite changed, and energy level drained to a point where everything you try to accomplish seems to require an overwhelming effort.

If headaches are gradually limiting your ability to function, you may find yourself facing ever-growing feelings of anxiety and depression. You may feel drawn into a downward spiral where the consequences of your headaches seem to cause even more headaches. If headaches dominate your life to this degree, seeing a counselor may be a necessary part of regaining some perspective for coping with these events.

If your headaches have resulted from an injury, the downward spiral of emotional distress may emerge long after the actual injury. This type of delayed reaction, sometimes called a *delayed grief reaction,* can be difficult to understand, but it usually makes sense. Immediately after the accident, the injured person is happy just to be alive and isn't surprised to experience some pain. But he or she anticipates that with healing the pain will also get better—if not within a few days, certainly within a few weeks. Sometimes, however, injuries that at first seemed minor can lead to pain that goes on and on. Each new visit to a doctor is initially a source of optimism, but as each new treatment effort proves not to work, frustration begins to rise. Eventually, friends, family, and especially employers and insurers, may begin to show signs of skepticism. They don't know what to make of all your pain, especially if nothing is broken or paralyzed. Weeks after the accident the future may seem much more uncertain than it did immediately after the accident. You may feel an ever-growing concern that the impact of the injury on your job, your marriage, or your leisure activities isn't going to end at some foreseeable time. With this uncertainty, plus the ongoing pain, feelings of helplessness, depression, and worry may become increasingly apparent.

Stressful Life Circumstances

There's no limit to the list of life circumstances that could be considered here. Consequently, stress researchers often try to divide the trials brought about by life's circumstances into those of *daily hassles* versus *prolonged stressors*.

Daily Hassles

Daily hassles are those ever-present little problems that can make your life so stressful. Often they are a matter of just not having enough time or resources to meet the challenges presented by the typical day. For a working parent this could mean getting up at a very early hour to get the kids off to school, and then getting yourself to work on time. Then, after a hectic day at work, rushing to pick up the children from daycare, stopping for groceries, and getting home in time to prepare an evening meal. Toss in a few unpredictable events, such as an illness, bad weather, or unreliable transportation, and the tension mounts quickly, the blood pressure rises, along with the familiar feeling of discomfort that begins to build in the temples, jaw, or back of the neck.

The big question concerning daily hassles is when should you just accept them as a normal part of life and try to control the resulting stress response, versus when is it time to seek ways to change the situations that produce the hassles? Sometimes you can think through this issue on your own; at other times, talking to a trusted friend or to a trained counselor might help you find some answers.

Prolonged Stressors

Some prolonged stressors might be intensified daily hassles that drag on for several days or weeks. Others might be more serious. At one time or another we have all encountered continuous, ongoing stressors with our jobs, finances, health, or personal relationships. Sometimes these can be so severe they nearly overwhelm us for months at a time, especially when no solution is in sight.

The problem with prolonged stressors is that they stay with us beyond the end of the workday. The worries go home with us; they can disrupt our sleep. The effects on our bodies are like those of a marathon run that never seems to end.

When faced with prolonged stress it's difficult to pinpoint whether today's headache is a result of a particular stressor. After all, the stressor was also present yesterday when you didn't have a headache. The danger is that you may fool yourself into believing that your headache therefore has nothing to do with the particular stressor. The truth of the matter regarding prolonged stressors is that they appear to lower our threshold for the onset of headaches. You just start to notice more headaches. A continuing stress also may increase your sensitivity to other common headache triggers.

If you have a significant amount of ongoing stress in your life, you can try to reduce the toll paid by your body by regular practice of self-regulating techniques. You should also try to identify and tackle the source of the stress. It can be really difficult to learn how to control your headaches when you are simultaneously feeling overwhelmed by other problems.

Personal Perception

One of the great mysteries of our lives and a source of constant intrigue to psychologists is how past experience shapes our reactions to the events of the present. This is especially true of our emotional reactions. Often, present emotional reactions appear to have a connection to past experience. This is most clearly seen with certain concrete fears. For example, if you nearly died from a snake bite at some time in the past, you probably still get anxious at the sight of a snake.

Most emotional links between the past and the present are much more subtle. For example, if you were physically, sexually, or emotionally mistreated as a child, feelings of depression and anxiety may surface more readily in response to the stressors of today. Thus, if you're trapped in an unsatisfactory relationship as an adult (or in any other type of situation that limits your functioning), feelings of despair may arise more readily than in someone with a more emotionally secure past. Headaches, like anything else that limits your personal autonomy, can leave you feeling trapped. They too can tie into personal perceptions, built on past experiences, which may amplify your feelings of suffering.

Certainly, individuals can overcome such traumatic past experiences by knowledge, self-reflection, and positive life experiences. Dealing with personal perceptions, however, can be difficult to do on your own. This is a dimension where professional counseling can be very helpful.

Personality Style as a Stressor

Closely related to personal perception are certain personality features long thought to be related to headaches, but never actually proven to be so. These features are compulsiveness, perfectionism, and impatience. It seems logical that a chronically impatient person, who always feels under pressure to get things done just right, may also experience a constantly heightened level of neuroendocrine arousal as a result of that pressure. His or her internal needs and perceptions may extract a physical price, by keeping the fight-or-flight response constantly simmering.

Of course, not all people with these personality characteristics have a problem with headaches, nor do all those who suffer from headaches have such personality traits. But this type of personality combined with a genetic predisposition for headaches may be a high risk combination. If you have headaches and find that you

- Are always the first to finish eating

- Are impatient when others don't talk fast enough

- Can't stand to wait in line

- Become irritated with tiny interruptions

- Make lists and set deadlines constantly—even at home

- Can't stand to leave your work unfinished even when you're tired

Then perhaps you should examine your philosophy of life. Why are you so intensely driven? Taking time to learn self-regulation relaxation techniques may help ease these personality traits that can function as constant stressors.

Counseling for Headaches

As with learning self-regulation, there's no single correct formula for helpful counseling. You must feel that the counselor understands you and that you can develop a trusting relationship with him or her. If you're seeking help from a psychotherapist for your headaches, it's important that you find someone knowledgeable about mind-body interactions, as well as the unique problems presented by headaches. Many psychologists, counselors, and social workers who provide counseling for dealing with personal stressors and perceptions also can assist you with learning the techniques of self-regulation.

The Power of Sharing

Just having someone willing to listen to you can be helpful. Recognizing your stressors, whether they are from your past, present, or future can be a useful place to start. Getting your bottled-up feelings off your chest can be a big relief. It can be very reassuring to know that your worries are an intrinsic part of your headache experience. You won't be the first person to discover that the stress of your life is taking a toll in the form of headaches; or that your headaches themselves are extracting a price from you emotionally. We must allow ourselves to recognize our lives are part of the human condition, and that for most people the human condition entails coping with suffering—whether the pain is physical or emotional.

Recent research by the psychologist James Pennebaker (1995) highlights the value of human communication in health maintenance. In a series of studies, people who were given opportunities to share troublesome concerns and secrets demonstrated over several months a lower rate of viral illness compared to control subjects without such opportunities. The increased neuroendocrine arousal caused by unexpressed emotion appears to suppress immune system functioning, which, in turn, lowers resistance to viral disease. Thus, immune compromise appears to be a critical physiological link between chronic stressors and health.

Addressing Control of Stressors

Sometimes you can become so embroiled in your daily hassles and/or prolonged stressors that you lose all sense of perspective. A neutral third party may be able to help you step back and think more objectively about the stressors in your life. What are they? Which ones should or shouldn't be tolerated? What are your options? What might be subject to change? What is within your power to change? How might you go about making these changes?

Bob's Story

Bob's case illustrates the value of changing those stressors that are within your reach. Bob was totally stressed out at work by negative feedback from his boss. His boss complained that Bob was frequently late for work, kept poor records, and didn't have the right personality for the job. Bob's workday got off to a poor start regularly because he had to drive through very heavy traffic. Stuck in lengthy traffic delays, he would become highly distressed because he knew his boss would criticize him for being late again. He frequently arrived at work with a headache that only got worse over the course of the day. Upon reflection, he decided that it wasn't wise to quit his job before he had another prospect. Quitting abruptly would just cause more stress for him and his family. In time, he acknowledged that with effort he could improve his tardiness and record keeping, but he also felt he couldn't do much about his boss not liking him. This seemed to be a realistic appraisal of his situation. His major stress reducer was quite a simple one; namely, to leave for work thirty minutes earlier in the morning to improve his chances of arriving on time. Making the behavioral change to get to work on time did actually improve the atmosphere for him at work because his day no longer started with a headache. He tried to ignore his perception that his boss didn't like him, and concentrated on other more positive aspects of his life. He also used self-regulation techniques at work for controlling both his negative feelings and his headaches. These efforts reduced his irritability at work and eventually the relationship with his boss improved. Certainly, the moral of this story is that Bob changed what he could, tried to accept what he couldn't, and thereby learned how to cope with stress in a much more effective way.

Addressing Personal Perceptions and Personality

There is still a lot of mystery associated with psychotherapy and often skepticism about the value of talking about one's past in order to cope with the problems of the present. Much of this skepticism is justified. Simply talking about the past, or finding someone in your past to blame for how you feel today, isn't going to magically change how well you function. Nonetheless, it can be useful to notice direct emotional links between your past and present and to use this knowledge to emotionally unhook your past from your present.

Consider in more detail how your reaction to headaches may be linked to your past emotional experience. A childhood that lacked basic security and nurturing can leave an adult with many unresolved feelings of anger, resentment, and depression. These negative emotions may appear to have been overcome by improved circumstances later in life. Job success and a good marriage can lead to enhanced emotional security and improved self-esteem. But, if many years later, this same person begins to experience severe headaches, there may be a reemergence of those feelings of anger, resentment, and depression. Such feelings are a natural reaction to the frustration created by headaches, but they may be further intensified by their experiential link to a past when there was little security or nurturing available. You could argue that such stirring of past emotions by headaches is irrational—but emotions are not logical. Headaches can expose emotional roots, which when uncovered can add to the suffering.

In fact, it's fairly common for people to report, in the throes of severe pain, the abrupt recollection of an unpleasant memory. Headaches, or any other severe pain, can do that to you. They can remind you of all the events in the past over which you had little control. Thus, shaped by your memories you react to the current headache episode with your unique personal perception. If you are experiencing this type of emotional "flashback" with your headaches, it's time for you to seek professional counseling. Most of us can learn some new behaviors to help us control some of the troublesome aspects of our personalities. In the case of traits that may be contributing to your headache proneness, even if you can't change the traits, you can certainly examine them and learn how to limit their negative consequences.

Additional Cognitive-Behavioral Coping Strategies

Here are some practical tips cognitive-behavioral counselors give to their clients for coping with the stressors that can bring on headaches.

Schedule a "Worry Time"

Sometimes it's useful to postpone worrisome thoughts and feelings. This doesn't mean that you should try to deny, ignore, or repress such concerns, but rather to have some choice about *when* you do your worrying. Being constantly preoccupied by worries makes you inefficient in your use of time. Such preoccupations can keep you from getting your work done and rob you of all pleasure from your daily routine. When you find yourself distracted by such thoughts, try using the following self-talk script:

✻ Script: To Stop Worrying

Stop! My worries are legitimate, but now isn't the time to be preoccupied. I have other things to do now. I will imagine taking that worry, putting it in a box, and slipping it into a drawer. I will then close the drawer and maybe even lock it. It will keep there just fine until I open the drawer during my "worry time."

Each day schedule as much time as you need—from a few minutes up to an hour or more—when you can open your worry drawer. Allow yourself to face your worries. If the worry is your headache or health, go ahead and explore your concerns. How do you feel about the changes in your life? What about your job, your finances, and/or your family? When your time is up, put the worries back in the drawer.

The rationale for the worry drawer is that when you have serious, realistic worries, it's meaningless simply to tell yourself "don't worry, don't be depressed, don't be frustrated." Such efforts often backfire, and the worrisome thought keeps sneaking back at inopportune times. It's human nature to worry, and sometimes worry does lead to problem solving. Instead, give your problems their due when you're ready. If you have ten minutes before an important appointment, a job to complete, or an exam—stop your worrisome thought for now, and put it in a drawer. Take the ten minutes to use your (BMW)I formula instead for a self-regulating exercise.

✻ Script: To Relax

Sit back, get comfortable, focus on your breathing, your muscles, and move to that calm/secure place in your mind—refresh your mind and body for ten minutes. Tell yourself, "Now isn't the time to tackle my deeper worries. Now is the time for a relaxation break to clear my head and restore my body for the task ahead."

Use a similar self-talk script if you find yourself waking up at night preoccupied with concerns. Three A.M. is seldom a productive time for problem solving. Rest and sleep should have a higher priority. If you absolutely must do your worrying in the middle of the night, go ahead and use that as your intentional worry time, but don't do it in bed. Get out of your bed, go to another room, and open up your worry drawer. When you're finished, close it up again. A bedroom should be for pleasurable experiences only—calm relaxation, intimacy, and sleep. Sleep is highly conditionable to its surroundings. Once you start doing too much worrying in bed, it can become a very bad habit.

Thought Stopping

Within the worry confinement suggestions above, you were also exposed to the idea of *thought stopping*. When thought stopping is needed, say or think:

✻ Script: For Thought Stopping

Stop! Stop that thought now! It's not a bad thought, but it is bad timing. I have more important things to do right now.

Pacing

If you must live with pain, *pacing* is an important concept. Runners in a race use the strategy of pacing themselves to avoid using up all of their energy too early in the race. Instead, they proceed at a pace that will produce their best time over the entire distance. Likewise, living with pain often means doing less now to get more done in the future. If you feel you must push yourself to the limit to complete a task today because you may be incapacitated with a headache tomorrow, it can become a self-fulfilling prophesy. Instead, if you pace yourself to permit a few brief (BMW)I breaks, you may get a little bit less done today but a lot more done tomorrow.

Keeping a Good/Bad List

Keep a written, or at least a mental, list of the good as well as the bad things in your life. Pull out this list when stressors and headaches seem overwhelming. No matter how bad things are, what is still good? The question, "Is my glass half empty or half full?" is a wise question to ask yourself. Of course, not every-one is dealt a great hand; in the game of life headaches don't abide by codes of fairness and justice. Nevertheless, what we choose to focus on can make a difference in how we feel. There are truly heroic individuals who, despite great physical and emotional pain, continue to live meaningful and productive lives.

Communicate Your Wishes

A lot of interpersonal "games" can arise when we have chronic pain or illness. Some people want attention, help, and sympathy; others do not. Don't leave your co-workers, friends, or loved ones guessing, "Why did he or she leave the room? Is he or she sick, angry, or distraught?" Make it clear to others how you prefer to deal with your headaches.

The extended family gathered for the holidays is a common example. If you're the host or hostess and have a headache and need assistance with dinner or housework, ask for it. Don't wait for people to notice how distressed you feel. Similarly, if you cope best by spending some time in a room by yourself, make it clear that's how you best handle a headache. It doesn't mean that you don't like your visitors or wish to blame them for your distress. You shouldn't turn a headache or any other physical problem into a game where others must guess what you want. If they guess wrong and you then feel justified in reminding them what sorry excuses they are for "caring" loved ones, you are playing a very dangerous manipulation game.

Accepting Is Not the Same as Forgetting

The process of adjustment to personal losses is frequently poorly understood. Even after the death of a loved one, well-meaning comforters may say or imply that you'll "forget" the loss in time. While it's true that the severity of emotional suffering will ease with time, it's not because you ever forget. What happens is that with the passage of time the memory becomes less painfully sharp. The same principle applies to loss of autonomy stemming from health problems, including headaches. If you previously enjoyed a daily walk, traveling, or physically active recreation, but now your health prevents this, you're not going to forget your loss. You'll never like it. Acceptance doesn't mean liking or forgetting—it means making adjustments.

Conclusion

The issues discussed above are a few examples of the types of strategies that can help you deal with the daily hassles, prolonged stressors, and personal perceptions that may have become part of your pattern of headaches. Be as honest with yourself as possible. If you have headaches and also feel depressed and miserable, is it just the headache pain? Or is it time to understand and try to alter some of those circumstances in your life that may be contributing to the cause of your headaches?

Key Word Summary

To ensure that you have thoroughly mastered the material in this chapter, write the definition of each term below in your own words.

Positive stressors: _____

_____

_____

Negative stressors: _____

_____

_____

Control of stressors: _____

_____

_____

Delayed grief reaction: _____

_____

_____

Daily hassles: _____

_____

_____

Prolonged stressors: _____

_____

_____

Past-present emotional link: _____

_____

_____

Personality traits as stressors: _____

_____

_____

Worry time: _____

_____

_____

Thought stopping: _____

_____

_____

Pacing: _____

_____

_____

Good/bad list: _____

_____

_____

Further Reading

Catalano, E. M. and K. N. Hardin. 1996. *The Chronic Pain Control Workbook*. Oakland, CA: New Harbinger Press.

Jamison, R. N. 1996. *Mastering Chronic Pain: A Professional's Guide to Behavioral Treatment*. Sarasota, FL: Professional Resource Press.

Meichenbaum, D. 1977. *Cognitive-Behavior Modification: An Integrative Approach*. New York: Plenum Press.

Chapter 10

Putting It All Together

▲ Headache management plan

▲ Key words and concepts of self-regulation

▲ An internal response image

▲ Patience, persistence, and positive attitude

▲ Some success stories

In this final chapter you can review your plan for managing your headaches. Understanding headaches, dealing with your doctor and medications, and recognizing the role of triggers are all important, but the focus of this workbook is learning self-regulation techniques. At this point you should know what to do, how to do it, and have confidence that this isn't an exotic magical strategy but simply a way to use the natural abilities of your body. Also, you should have a sense of how self-regulation applies to all three aspects of headache control—*prevention* of headache, *reduction* of severity, and *tolerance* when necessary.

Your Headache Management Plan Overview

1. Decide whether you need to see a doctor, or whether you can handle your headaches on your own. You must check with a doctor if

   • Your headache symptoms suddenly change for the worse

   • You're using too much nonprescription medication

   • You're using other people's pain medication

   • Your headaches are interfering with your daily activities

2. If your headaches require medication, make sure you have a plan worked out with your doctor about when and how to use medications

   • Emergency room treatment alone is an inadequate plan

   • Be alert to when medications may be contributing to your headache cycle

   • Recognize differences between medications for immediate relief versus medications for prevention of headaches

3. Avoid food and airborne headache triggers as best you can

   • Know your triggers, but don't become obsessed with them

   • Be on the lookout for trigger interactions

4. Keep yourself as physically fit as possible

   • A fit body recovers from stress faster

   • A fit body is less likely to be harmed by stress

5. Pay particularly close attention to the conditioning, posture, and relaxation of the muscles of your upper back, neck, and jaw

   • Tension tends to find its way into these muscles

   • You can be unaware of tension until you feel pain

6. Pay close attention to the activation level of your autonomic/neuroendocrine system. Tension is expressed in

   • Cold clammy hands

   • Rapid heart rate, shortness of breath, knot in your stomach

   • Feeling on edge, restless, inability to concentrate

7. Learn and practice cognitive-physiological self-regulation as outlined in the Scan, Focus, (BMW)I plan

   • Cognitive means your mind—your internal awareness, your mind's TV screen

   • Physiological means your body—your nervous system, muscles, organs, and glands

8. Keep a headache log to

   • Help you monitor pattern of headaches and interactions with triggers, stressors, and mood

   • Help you monitor setbacks and progress

9. Recognize your stressors (both daily hassles and prolonged stressors)

   • Avoid or change those stressors that you can

   • Seek counseling if stressors seem out of control

   • Be sensitive to personal perceptions and personality traits that may add to your level of stress

Key Words and Concepts of Self-Regulation

1. Your *brain activation level* can amplify pain sensations up or turn them down. That's why relaxation techniques can lower your awareness of pain.

2. Your *physical functions* and sensations follow your brain's lead. That is why imagination via focused attention can lower physical activation and pain.

3. *Pain is a neurologic alarm signal to the brain*, and a headache can be among the loudest of alarms. Imagination, via focused attention, can provide the brain with competing signals.

It's sometimes helpful to take a slip of paper, or a 3" x 5" card, to use as your cue guide when you practice. Write on the card:

SCAN—FOCUS—(BMW)I

Or you could put together a more elaborate cueing outline, such as

Scan for cognitive and physical signs of tension and early warning signs of a headache.

Focus attention on

- Imagining the "calm/relax" wall with gate

- Letting the gate open to a peaceful, serene, safe scene

- Beginning your focus on the building blocks

(BMW)I—the building blocks of self-regulation:

B: Slow, deep diaphragmatic breathing

M: Let all the tension out of your muscles starting with your jaw; feel the heaviness

W: Feel the warmth flowing into your hands

Ia: Imagine the feelings above and add supportive images

Ib: Try creating images that directly compete with pain

Maximum: Full-scale (BMW)I self-regulation session, requiring ten to twenty minutes in a quiet place in a comfortable chair or bed.

Minimum: Whatever you can do wherever you are. Take a few slow, deep breaths and start with your jaw to let all the tension out.

Partial Relaxation: Relaxing muscles in parts of your body, even while the rest of your muscles remain in use.

Developing an Internal Response Image

Part of successfully acquiring relaxation skills is to develop what has been referred to as a relaxation "response image," i.e., the subjective experience you feel as your muscles relax, your heart rate and blood pressure drop, your hands feel warmer, and your mind clears. Once you recognize that internal feeling, it'll become easier for you to reproduce it quickly in a wide variety of circumstances. At that point, you truly will have developed an effective stress and pain-management coping skill.

Acquiring this response image can be compared to the learning of other skills. At first, learning to hit a golf or tennis ball can seem very challenging. There is too much to think about: the position of your hands, arms, feet, torso, head, etc. Then, there are all the angles and arcs to think about. But eventually with practice, it can all come together resulting in a certain "feel" for the swing without requiring conscious thought about all the individual elements that make up the complex motor movement. This too will also happen with self-regulation eventually. You will scan nearly automatically. Focus on a few slow-deep breaths, and almost instantly you will feel the tension release and warmth sweeping through your body, most noticeably in your jaw, neck, chest, and hands.

A clear internal response image is the last step for controlling your reflexive flight-or-fight response and thus becoming a calmer, more relaxed, less headache-prone person. Now, when you feel the inevitable stress reaction, it can be your cue to "let go" and replace the stress reaction with the feeling of calmness. Even if you don't feel internally calm, go ahead and relax your body—use a *minimum* or *partial* relaxation technique if that is all that time or circumstances will permit. I believe that many people who appear to be calm in stressful or pressured situations have learned to do this. They know how to let go of the tension in their body and how to keep their attention focused. Athletes who perform well under pressure and students who perform well on tests are common examples. Such individuals have many of the same anxieties as the rest of us, but they have learned to let go of tension and to focus on the task at hand.

Barriers to Learning Self-Regulation for Headaches

If self-regulation techniques are as useful in controlling headaches as research suggests they are, why doesn't everyone use them? The most common reason is that most people are unaware of such techniques. Others may be vaguely aware, but believe that these are highbrow activities for those with a New Age philosophy of life. Fortunately, many people have developed effective self-regulation relaxation skills, without ever having identified them as such. But even for those presented with the opportunity to learn self-regulation training, there are common attitudes and beliefs in our culture that can get in their way. Some of the more common obstacles I have encountered include the following:

"I Want Instant Relief"

In the throes of a full-blown migraine the desire for instant relief is understandable. The suffering person wants self-regulation to work like a narcotic painkiller. Unfortunately, self-regulation exercises seldom provide such quick pain relief. It takes time and practice to learn to use self-regulation. Any benefits for headaches can be very slow to accrue. The process of acquiring a skill is quite different from taking a pill. If you learn to self-regulate your headaches to any significant degree, you will have accomplished something of lasting value. You will have learned to control a basic physiological reaction, which in time can lead to fewer headaches. By contrast, pain pills can provide only symptomatic relief

Of course, there are exceptions to the statements above. I have seen individuals who, after developing an awareness of the link between tightening the jaw and tension headaches, never experienced a tension headache again. But this is the rare exception, especially for those with long-standing headache problems.

"I Tried It Once and It Didn't Help Me"

An all too common scenario is that as headaches escalate, doctors, family, or the person with the pain begin to worry about the increasing dependency on medication. At this point, a health care worker, friend, or family member may mention the need to reduce stress and may provide the headache sufferer with a cassette tape with relaxation instructions and the mandate "try this." With the next migraine attack, the pain-engulfed person "tries" to listen to the tape, but experiences no headache relief and concludes, "It doesn't work for me." Similarly, the headache sufferer in the midst of a week-long migraine may come to a therapist from the ER with a referral for "biofeedback." The results are equally futile.

Such one-shot attempts at self-regulation are like a novice tennis player taking a twenty-minute tennis lesson and becoming disillusioned when he or she can't play like a pro. Acquiring *any* skill takes practice, time, and patience.

"I Don't Have the Time to Practice"

All this talk about lessons and practice may sound like just one more item to add to an already hectic, time-pressured schedule. But take the time, and you'll be surprised. We find time to do the things that are important to us. You may end up with more time rather than less. Think of all the lost time and lost efficiency caused by your headaches. Improvement in focusing your attention alone can improve efficiency at a variety of tasks. Take the time to learn to use (BMW)I self-regulation and you'll never be sorry. I have never met anyone who improved their ability to self-regulate who regretted the time spent.

"It Just Seems Too Complicated"

Another version of "It's too complicated" is "I'm a practical person, just give me a pill for my headache." In some cases this may be a mask for the discomfort of doing something so "psychological." In other cases, however, self-regulation may indeed seem unduly complicated when you begin to explore the various methods and schools of thought on teaching self-regulation.

Remember that the array of self-regulation techniques is less different than you might suppose, and that it's the common elements of focusing attention and somatic relaxation that have a great deal to do with the positive benefits of all the techniques. That is why one of the goals of this workbook is to provide a structure of simple building blocks.

Still another reason for self-regulation seeming too complicated is having an overcompulsive concern about doing it "just right." If your headache isn't instantly relieved, it doesn't mean you're doing something wrong. The paradox here is that, although there is some virtue in doing things in a structured way, it may be that this internal goal of compulsive perfectionism is a personal stressor that's part of your headache syndrome. Hopefully, this workbook conveys a happy medium. There are things that you must learn and practice, but very little of self-regulating is a matter of doing it correctly. It's a frame of reference more than an absolute standard.

"Maybe It Works for Others, but My Headaches ..."

You can finish that sentence however you wish. "Need real medicine" probably fills in the blank most often. Instead of self-regulation techniques being too complicated, they are too simple. Some individuals feel insulted when they are told that merely focusing on their breathing and relaxing their muscles could possibly affect headaches as complicated and profound as theirs are.

When I hear this objection I am reminded of an Old Testament story. A rich potentate from a foreign country suffering from leprosy came to the prophet Elijah and promised him many great gifts if he would cure him of his leprosy. Elijah refused the gifts and told the ruler simply to go and bathe in the river Jordan. The ruler, having expected to be put to a much more exotic test than swimming in a dirty river, went away highly miffed. He reconsidered only after his humble servant reminded him that if the prophet had made some outrageously difficult demand, he would have done all he could to fulfill it. Thus prodded, he visited the river and was healed. Maybe (BMW)I self-regulation can be your river Jordan.

"It Works When You Do It, But Not When I Try It Myself"

Every teacher of self-regulation techniques has heard this line. It's true that when you're just starting, it's easier to focus your attention when someone else is guiding you. For that reason, making tapes from the scripts included in this workbook or purchasing commercially available cassette tapes can be helpful. But remind yourself that you're always doing it yourself no matter who is talking. If you experience cognitive-physiological changes, *you* did it—it's your mind and body. Even with biofeedback, the sensors and wires are monitoring only what you are doing—they're not doing anything to you.

At the heart of this problem, I believe, is a lack of confidence in knowing what to do. Hopefully, the simple building block approach described in this workbook can provide you with the necessary belief that you do know what to do.

"It's Against My Religion"

Religious beliefs must always be respected. However, this objection, I suspect, is based on a flat-out misconception of what self-regulation is. How can learning to become more relaxed and better control one's pain possibly be a violation of any particular religion?

Seemingly this concern arises from the misconception that focused attention, because of its similarity to meditation, is an Eastern religious practice that has been adopted by New Age religions. Therefore, to some, learning self-regulation represents the worship of a false god. Given my personal involvement with a traditional Western religion, I find this thinking particularly disconcerting. Focused attention, and using focused attention for physiological self-regulation, is not the unique province of any particular religious tradition anymore than running and jumping is the province of any particular culture. It's like saying that thinking, breathing, or letting my heart beat is against my beliefs.

The Three P's of Coping: Patience, Persistence, and Positive Attitude

Most headaches reflect a well-established pattern of muscular and neurohormonal responses that have developed and become habitual over many years. Don't expect to alter such patterns easily or rapidly. It may take weeks or even months before you notice significant changes in your headaches, even after you have acquired the fundamental relaxation skills. An early positive sign can be any change in the pattern of the headache suggesting that you're doing something that is beginning to disrupt well-entrenched physical responses. Your early warning signs may change somewhat, or the headache itself may occur at a different time of the day. Since positive improvement may be gradual, it can be useful for you to keep careful records of the intensity, frequency, and duration of your headaches.

Because you can't judge the success of your self-regulation solely on whether or not you have a headache today, it's important to keep a record. Only in a log that reflects many months of headache activity will you see whether you actually have been able to prevent headaches, reduce their severity when they occur, or at least improve your emotional tolerance of the full-blown ones that remain.

You can only do so much with your efforts, and then you must let nature take its course. With self-regulation you're trying to work *with* your body rather than against it. The mental attitude required to achieve hand warming can be considered symbolic of the entire spirit of self-regulating headaches. You can't actually "make" your hands warm, anymore than you can "make" your headaches disappear. The harder you try to make your hands warm, the cooler they will become. *You can only allow it to happen.* You can only *imagine* warmth flowing into your hands. If you can "feel" it in your imagination, you have done all you can. Only nature will determine if your hands will follow. In the long run, patience, persistence, and a positive attitude will permit nature to be on your side.

Some Headache Control Success Stories

I will conclude by describing three individuals whom I have had the privilege of assisting with headache control. These cases illustrate some of the differences in headache patterns outlined in chapter 1 and show the wide range of headache problems that can benefit from the development of self-regulation skills. Although these stories are true, the names, of course, have been changed.

Larry: Occasional (Episodic) Mild to Moderate Headache

Larry's headaches represent the type of pattern most likely to respond quickly to self-regulation training and most likely to be completely controlled with self-regulation alone.

When I first saw Larry he was a thirty-one-year-old sales representative for a metal products company. He was energetic, extroverted, doing well as a salesman and rising in his company. He had been married for five years and had two young children. The marriage appeared to be stable and happy. He reported having noticed tension headaches in certain situations for at least the past ten years. His first memory of a headache was while he was in college during his final exams. Presently, headaches had begun to crop up while he was driving long distances or involved in a major sales presentation or negotiation. His concern about his headaches increased with his success in the company because of growing demands for more regional travel and more major presentations.

His headache symptoms clearly fell into the tension category. He could continue to work with a headache but found it very unpleasant. He also expressed a vague concern about too much reliance on alcohol to feel relaxed. Except for his headache complaint, he was a healthy, physically fit young man who was happy with his life.

Larry learned the basic (BMW)I skills very quickly. After only a few days of practice he reported feeling that he nearly could completely control his headache symptoms. More specifically he began to notice that when he was driving, the first hint of pain was a slight tightening and tinge of discomfort just above and forward of the tops of his ears (presumably in the fan-shaped temporalis muscle). Briefly concentrating on letting his jaw become relaxed and slack seemed to stop the discomfort.

He still felt tense before a presentation, but by focusing on breathing and a quick muscle tension review he could control his tension. Nearly fifteen years later, I happened to see him in a supermarket and he told me that he had never experienced another significant headache after he learned how to do these relaxation "tricks."

I realize that if you have serious migraine you may ask, "How bad could Larry's problems really have been compared to mine?" While that is certainly a legitimate question, the point is there are millions of people who suffer periodic minor headaches who could eliminate them entirely with just a little knowledge about the physiology of headaches and a little practice using the very simple principles of mind/body interaction.

Beth: Occasional (Episodic) Severe Headaches

Beth is typical of the most prevalent of all headache types that turn up in the office of a primary care physician.

Beth was thirty-nine years old when I first met her. She recalled having had migraine headaches from the time she was thirteen or fourteen. For many years they seemed to be menstrual migraines, appearing on the day, or a day or two before, her period began. Often she could ignore them, sometimes she took aspirin, and if the attack was really severe, she would stay home from school. This pattern continued through her college years, during the early years of her subsequent marriage, and during her career as a middle-school teacher and administrator. With the added responsibilities of a career and family, however, she no longer had the luxury of staying home on a bad headache day. She began to rely increasingly on medication to keep functioning. Most medications seemed to help at first, but slowly they would lose their effectiveness.

Beth and her husband separated after nearly twenty years of marriage. This was a difficult time for her, compounded by the stresses associated with her now being the principal of her school. Her headaches escalated out of control and she was referred to me for self-regulation training by her primary care physician, who continued to manage her medication. Like Larry she was highly motivated to get her headaches under control and regularly practiced her (BMW)I exercises when stressed and for her headaches. We also spent some time talking about her life stressors. She instituted a number of changes to reduce her stress at work and to resolve her uncertain marital status. Additionally, she had several visits with a physical therapist who helped her develop a set of exercises for improving the posture, strength, and flexibility of her neck muscles.

Progress for Beth was much slower than for Larry, but within a few weeks she noted a trend toward less severe headaches. Gradually she required less medication, and eventually she reported a decrease in the frequency of her headaches. She was particularly enthusiastic about her success one day when at the first sign of a migraine she locked the door of her office, took twenty minutes to achieve a state of profound relaxation, and the headache never developed.

Between careful use of medication, exercise, and self-regulation, Beth now feels that she has adequate control of her headaches. Her experience is a classic example of how physiological predisposition and life stresses can gradually combine into a serious escalating headache pattern. But with effort it is a pattern that can be broken.

Elaine: Frequent Severe Headaches, Sometimes Continuous for Weeks

Elaine represents an atypical headache case, but her story is not unfamiliar to those headache specialists who see highly complex refractory cases.

Like Beth, Elaine's headaches started in early adolescence. In addition to her headaches, unfortunately, she had to contend with a highly dysfunctional family. She was the only daughter of a father who drank excessively and had little respect for women. When Elaine was thirteen her mother died, leaving her with a father who behaved more like a demanding, helpless adolescent than a father. After her mother's death, Elaine seldom went to school. While her father and her brothers hunted, fished, and went to work, Elaine was left at home to do the domestic chores. Sexual abuse was also part of the sordid pattern, although not from immediate family members. From age thirteen until her mid-twenties she had almost no social or personal life beyond the family home.

During these years of isolation, Elaine's headaches evolved into a nearly constant mixed headache pattern, in which she always had a tension headache frequently compounded by migraines. Periodically, she would develop a massive unrelenting headache that would continue for days on end. At such times she would say that she just wanted to die. At least twice she was hospitalized following a pill overdose. Overdosing seemed to be her only means of protest. It certainly captured the attention of her father and brothers. By the time I first saw her there had been multiple psychiatric and neurological hospitalizations following attacks that could last for weeks at a time.

Too often with cases like Elaine's, an inordinate dependency and demand for medication (often narcotic analgesics) becomes part of the presenting pattern. Surprisingly, the first time I saw her she seemed remarkably disinterested in medication and expressed a strong interest in learning self-regulation techniques. Most of all she just seemed to want someone to talk to about her terrible life circumstances.

The course of her recovery was not rapid or easy, but in time it was remarkably complete. It included an almost religious-like allegiance to self-regulation techniques and some profound changes in her behavior. These changes ultimately led Elaine to become more independent. She began to express her anger about her family, and she got a job away from home. As she became more independent, she noted many maneuvers on the part of her father and brothers to interfere with her life. Part of her recovery was also learning to manage her medication more responsibly. She learned to use medication as part of her plan for headache control, rather than as a tool for manipulation.

There Is Hope for Headache Sufferers

If you have problems with headaches, you can probably fit yourself somewhere in the spectrum between Larry and Elaine—hopefully closer to Larry's case. But no matter where you fit, there is hope. Between your own effort and, if necessary, supported by the guidance of a knowledgeable doctor or other headache therapist, there is hope. No one should suffer the way Elaine suffered, or feel as distressed as Beth, or even feel as inconvenienced as Larry. I wish you well in your efforts to obtain control over your headaches and sincerely hope the information contained in this book is of value to you.

Appendix:
More Muscle Relaxation Scripts

Active Muscle Relaxation

The active form of muscle relaxation comes from the tradition of Progressive Muscle Relaxation (PMR) developed by Edmund Jacobson in the 1920s (1974). PMR training makes extensive use of "tense-relax" exercises in which you focus attention on tightening up a muscle, or muscle group, and then note the contrasting sensation as you release the tension. The goal is to help you increase your awareness of how a tense muscle feels compared to a relaxed muscle. For those who have difficulty with the passive letting go of muscle tension, this is a particularly useful approach. It gives you something very concretely physical to do while you are acquainting yourself with the process of muscle relaxation.

Take about ten to twenty minutes once or twice a day to focus on these four muscle groups. Work for two days on each muscle group before moving on to the next one. Begin by lying down or sitting in a comfortable chair with your head supported (see figure A.1). Take several deep breaths, releasing each breath slowly. Once slow-deep breathing has been established, let that be your cue to begin your muscle relaxation session.

Note: Contract the muscles as stated in the script as much as you can, but if you experience soreness do not strain or overdo it.

✱ <u>Script</u>: Muscle Group 1

  1. *Focus on the first group of muscles—your right hand, arm, and biceps. Make a fist, clenching as hard as you can. Hold that tension, feeling it creep up*

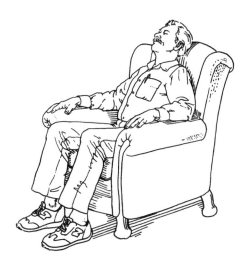

Figure A.1:   **Seated, Relaxed Position to Increase Breath and Muscle Awareness**

your arm toward your shoulder. Hold it until you begin to feel a slight cramping, burning sensation.

2. *Now relax, feeling all the tense muscles go limp. Feel the warming blood flow through your arm into your hand and fingers. Notice the contrast between what your muscles felt like when they were tense and what they feel like now that they are relaxed.*

3. *Repeat this procedure twice. Remember to pay attention to your breathing as you tense and relax. Does your breathing begin to get shallow when you tense? Make sure you do not hold your breath unconsciously.*

4. *Now notice how your right arm and hand feel in comparison to your left arm and hand. Now focus on your left hand, arm, and biceps and repeat the same exercise three times.*

After working for two days on the first muscle group, move on to the second group: feet, calves, thighs, and buttocks. Repeat the same procedure as above, alternating sides of your body.

✱ Script: Muscle Group 2

1. *Focus on your right foot and calf. Tighten them as hard as you can. You can either pull your foot upward, or stretch your foot outward by pointing your toe. Hold the tension, feeling it creep up your leg toward your torso. Hold the tension until you begin to feel a slight cramping, burning, sensation.*

2. *Now relax and feel the muscles go limp. Feel the warming blood flow through your calf and foot. Notice the contrast between what your muscles felt like when you were tense and what they feel like now that you are relaxed.*

3. *Repeat this procedure twice. Remember to pay attention to your breathing as you tense and relax. Does your breathing begin to get shallow? Make sure you're not holding your breath unconsciously.*
4. *Now notice how your right calf and foot feel compared to your left calf and foot. Focus on your left calf and foot and repeat the exercise three times.*
5. *Now focus on your right leg again. Tense your thigh and buttocks as you tense your foot and calf. Tense as hard as you can, until you begin to feel a slight cramping and burning sensation.*
6. *Now relax, feeling all the muscles in your right leg go limp. Feel the warming blood flow through your buttocks, thigh, calf, and foot. Notice the contrast between what your leg felt like when it was tense and what it feels like now that it is relaxed.*
7. *Repeat this procedure twice. Remember to do relaxed and natural breathing. Notice how your right leg feels compared to your left leg.*
8. *Now focus on your left leg, tensing your buttocks and thigh as you tense your left foot and calf. Repeat the exercise three times.*

After two days of working with muscle group 2, begin your practice on the third group of muscles: chest, stomach, and lower back.

* Script: Muscle Group 3

1. *Focus on your chest, stomach, and lower back. Tense those areas, lightly pushing your lower back into the bed or chair as you contract your abdominal muscles and shrug your shoulders. Hold the tension until you begin to feel a slight cramping, burning sensation.*
2. *Now relax, feeling your muscles go limp. Feel the warming blood flow through your lower back, stomach, and chest. Notice the contrast between how these areas felt when they were tense and what they feel like now.*
3. *Repeat this procedure twice. Remember to do relaxed and natural breathing.*

After two days, begin your practice on the fourth muscle group. For the next two days, focus on your shoulder, neck, throat, face, and head muscles. Pay special attention to your face, jaw, and throat, because the muscles in these areas are extremely sensitive to stress and anxiety and they may often be tense without you realizing it.

* Script: Muscle Group 4

1. *Focus first on your shoulder muscles. Do a "shoulder shrug" by raising your shoulders as close to your ears as possible. Hold it. Feel the knots begin to form in the trapezius muscles and back of your neck. Now relax your shoulder muscles. Feel the difference when these muscles are at rest and smooth, rather than tensed up.*

2. *Now turn your attention to your head. Wrinkle your forehead as tight as you can. Now relax and smooth it. Imagine your entire forehead and scalp becoming smooth and at rest. Now frown and notice the strain spreading throughout your forehead. Let go. Allow your brow to become smooth again. Now close your eyes tightly and squint. Feel the tension. Relax your eyes. Let them remain closed, gently and comfortably. Now clench your jaw, bite hard, and notice the tension throughout your jaw. Relax your jaw. When your jaw is relaxed, your lips should be slightly parted. Let yourself really appreciate the contrast between tension and relaxation. Now press your tongue against the roof of your mouth. Feel the ache in the back of your mouth. Relax. Now press your lips together and purse them into an "O." Relax your lips. Notice that your forehead, scalp, eyes, jaw, tongue, and lips are all relaxed.*

Differential Relaxation

Differential relaxation is an important variation of progressive muscle relaxation. You still tense and relax as you would with regular PMR, but you tense and relax different groups at the same time. Here is an example:

✳ Script: Differential Relaxation

Start with tensing your right hand and arm, while keeping your left arm as relaxed as possible. Then switch your tense versus relaxed sides. Do the same with your feet, calves, thighs, and buttocks. An even greater challenge is to tense-relax diagonal muscle groups. For example, tense your right arm and hand at the same time that you tense your left thigh, leg, and foot; then let go and relax. While one diagonal muscle group is tense, focus on keeping the diagonal muscle group relaxed. Then switch.

There is an important principle behind differential relaxation. The principle is that while some muscles are tense, others can still be relaxed. It's similar to squeezing one eye tightly, then opening it and squeezing the other, etc., over and over. This is important in daily life where some muscles must be in use while you walk, stand, or work at your desk, but others can remain relaxed. It doesn't aid your driving to have your entire body tensed when all you need is light tension to maintain your sitting posture, and occasional tension in your hands and arms to steer, and in your feet to control floor pedals.

Passive Muscle Relaxation

As you can probably guess, rather than tensing and then relaxing, passive muscle relaxation (sometimes called "release-only" relaxation) focuses just on the tension-release aspect of muscle relaxation. Once you thoroughly recognize how different a relaxed muscle feels from a tensed muscle, there may be no need for you to tense first. Passive muscle relaxation is also frequently associated with Autogenic

Training, a technique for focusing attention on muscle relaxation and warming at the same time.

✻ Script: Passive Muscle Relaxation—Release-Only

1. *Sit in a comfortable chair with your arms at your side and move around a bit until you're comfortable.*

2. *Begin to focus on your breathing. Breathe in deeply and feel the pure air fill your stomach, your lower chest, and your upper chest. Hold your breath for a moment as you sit up straighter, and then breathe out slowly through your mouth, feeling all tension and worry blow out in a stream. After you've exhaled completely, relax your stomach and your chest. Continue to take full, calm, even breaths, noticing that you become more relaxed with each breath.*

3. *Now relax your forehead, smoothing out all the lines. Keep breathing deeply . . . and then relax your eyebrows. Just let all the tension melt away, all the way down to your jaw. Let it all go. Now let your lips separate and relax your tongue. Breathe in and breathe out and relax your throat. Notice how soft and loose your entire face feels.*

4. *Roll your head gently and feel your neck relax. Release your shoulders. Just let them drop all the way down. Your neck is loose, and your shoulders are heavy and low. Now let the relaxation travel down through your arms to your fingertips. Your arms are heavy and loose. Your mouth is slightly open because your jaw is relaxed, too.*

5. *Breathe in deeply and feel your abdomen expand and then your chest. Hold your breath for a moment and then breathe out slowly in a smooth stream through your mouth.*

6. *Let the feeling of relaxation spread to your stomach. Feel all the muscles in your abdomen release their tension as it assumes its natural shape. Relax your waist and relax your back. Continue to breath deeply. Notice how loose and heavy the upper half of your body feels.*

7. *Now relax the lower half of your body. Feel your buttocks sink into the chair. Relax your thighs. Relax your knees. Feel the relaxation travel through your calves to your ankles, to the bottoms of your feet, all the way down to the tips of your toes. Your feet feel warm and heavy on the floor in front of you. With each breath, feel the relaxation deepen.*

8. *Now scan your body for tension as you continue to breathe. Your legs are relaxed. Your back is relaxed. Your shoulders and arms are relaxed. Your face is relaxed. There's a strong feeling of peace and warmth and relaxation.*

9. *If any muscle felt hard to relax, turn your attention to it now. Is it your back? Your thighs? Your jaw? Tune into the muscle and now tense it. Hold it tighter and release. Feel it join the rest of your body in a deep, deep relaxation.*

Your final goal is to be able to get fully relaxed in about a five-to-seven-minute session with these release-only strategies.

Autogenic Phrases

Still another form of passive muscle relaxation uses autogenic phrases. This is the use of simple repetitive phrases that suggest a certain feeling in the body. Their simplicity makes these phrases easy to memorize, and the repetitiveness encourages the body to follow the sensations on which the mind is focused. As you know by now, the choice to focus attention on the physical sensations of *heaviness* and *warmth* is not chosen randomly. Feelings of heaviness correspond to muscle relaxation and warmth to hand warming.

Repeat (or think to yourself) the verbal formulas below for two to ten minutes several times a day. Each time you say a phrase, say it slowly, taking about five seconds, and then pause for about three seconds. Repeat each phrase three or four times. Allow yourself to feel the sensations as you repeat each phrase softly to yourself or think it in your mind. You can go at your own pace. You may wish to begin with a day or two of just working on your arms before you move onto your arms and legs.

✱ Script: Autogenic Muscle Relaxation

My right arm is heavy.
My left arm is heavy.
Both of my arms are heavy.
My right leg is heavy.
My left leg is heavy.
My arms and legs are heavy.
My right arm is heavy.
Both of my arms are heavy.
Both of my legs are heavy.
My arms and legs are heavy.

Which Is Better—Active or Passive Muscle Relaxation?

Each type has its place. When just getting started, the active tense-relax exercise has the advantage of being a set of very concrete movements to perform. The effort involved focuses attention and immediately highlights the important contrast between a tense and a relaxed muscle. Note that some people who are chronically tense initially have trouble making this distinction.

The passive techniques allow for reaching a deeper level of absolute relaxation. The tense-relax technique periodically reactivates muscles, which activates the ANS, and the ANS regulates the cardiovascular system. Once you clearly recognize the difference between tension and relaxation in all the targeted muscle groups, you may prefer passive techniques because they will allow you to approach that ideal physiological state where muscle tension and physical activity drop so low, the body feels as if it were asleep. Your mind is still attentive.

References and Additional Reading

Bakal, D. A. 1994. *The Psychobiology of Chronic Headache*. New York: Springer Publishing Co.

Bakal, D. A., S. Demjen, and P.N. Duckro. 1994. "Chronic daily headache and the elusive nature of somatic awareness." In *Psychological Vulnerability to Chronic Pain*. Edited by R. C. Grzesiak and D. S. Ciccone. New York: Springer Publishing Co.

Blanchard, E. B. and S. Diamond. 1996. "Psychological treatment of benign headache disorders." *Professional Psychology: Research and Practice* 27: 541–547.

Drevets, W. C., H. Burton, T. O. Videen, A. Z. Snyder, J. R. Simpson, and M. E. Raichle. 1995. "Blood flow changes in human somatosensory cortex during anticipated stimulation." *Nature* 373, 249–252.

Hatch, J. P. 1993. "Headache." In *Psychophysiological Disorders: Research and Clinical Applications*. Edited by R. J. Gatchel and E. B. Blanchard. Washington, D.C.: American Psychological Association. 111–149.

Hatch, J. P., P. J. Moore, M. Cyr-Provost, N. N. Boutros, E. Seleshi, and S. Borcherding. 1992. "The use of electromyography and muscle palpation in the diagnosis of tension-type headache with and without pericranial muscle involvement." *Pain* 49: 175–178.

Jacobsen, Edmund. 1974. *Progressive Relaxation*. Chicago: The University of Chicago Press, Midway reprint.

Langemark, M., K. Jensen, T. S. Jensen, and J. Olesen. 1989. "Pressure pain thresholds and thermal nociceptive thresholds in chronic tension-type headache." *Pain* 38: 203–210.

Louis, I. and J. Olesen. 1982. "Evaluation of pericranial tenderness and oral function in patients with common migraine, muscle contraction headache and combination headache." *Pain* 12: 385–393.

Matthew, N. T. 1981. "Prophylaxis of migraine and mixed headache: A randomized controlled study." *Headache* 21: 105–109.

National Institutes of Health Technology Assessment Statement. 1995. "Integration of behavioral and relaxation approaches into the treatment of chronic pain and insomnia." Oct. 19-28, 1–34.

Olesen, J. 1991. "Clinical and pathophysiological observations in migraine and tension-type headache explained by integration of vascular, supraspinal, and myofascial inputs." *Pain* 46: 125–132,

Pennebaker, James W. (Ed.) 1995. *Emotion, Disclosure and Health.* Washington, D.C.: American Psychological Association.

Selye, Hans. 1956. *The Stress of Life.* New York: Mcgraw-Hill.

Resources

The organizations, publications, and products listed below may help you to obtain more information and help for your headaches.

Organizations

The most comprehensive source of general information on headaches is

The National Headache Foundation
428 St. James Place
Second Floor
Chicago, IL 60614-2750
(800) 843-2256; (312) 388-6399
Fax: (312) 525-7357
http://www.headaches.org

Other useful sources for information include

American Council for Headache Education (ACHE)
875 Kings Highway
Suite 200
Woodbury, NJ 08096-3172
(609) 348-8760

American Pain Society
4700 W. Lake Avenue
Glenview, IL 60025-4777
(847) 375-4715

The Migrane Association of Canada
365 Bloor Street
Suite 1912
Toronto, Ontario

Canada M4W 3L4
(800) 663-3357; (416) 920-4916
http://www.migrane.ca

World Cervicogenic Headache Society
c/o Rothbart Pain Management Clinic
16 York Mills Road
Unit 125, Box 129
North York, Ontario
Canada M2P 2E5
(416) 512-6407

"Headache Central" is the Web site of the Michigan Headache Treatment Network. http://www.medsupport.com/headache/index.html

"Migraine Resource Center" is the Web site of the Glaxo Wellcome Pharmaceutical Co. http://www.migrainehelp.com

Publications

APS Bulletin
C. Richard Chapman, Ph.D., Editor
American Pain Society
4700 W. Lake Avenue
Glenview, IL 60025-1485
(847) 375-4715

Biofeedback
Donald Moss, Ph.D., Editor
Association for Applied Psychophysiology and Biofeedback
10200 West 44th Avenue, No. 304
Whead Ridge, CO 80033-2842

Biofeedback and Self-Regulation
Frank Andrasik, Ph.D., Editor
Center for Behavioral Medicine
University of West Florida
11000 University Parkway
Pensacola, FL 32514-5751

The Clinical Journal of Pain
Peter R. Wilson, Ph.D., Editor-in-Chief
Mayo Clinic
200 First Street SW
Rochester, MN 55905

Journal of Psychotherapy
Wade H. Silverman, Ph.D., Editor
P. O. Box 330158
Miami, FL 33233-0158
(305) 854-0848

Mind/Body Medicine
Richard Friedman, Ph.D., Co-Editor-in-Chief
Department of Psychiatry
Building C, South Campus, Room 177
State University of New York
Stony Brook, NY 11794-8790
(516) 632-8845

Products

4-in-1 WAL-PIL-O
RoLoKe Co.
5760 Hannum Avenue
Culver City, CA 90231
(800) 533-8212

Posture Curve Lumbar Pillow
BodyCare, Inc.
Box 219
315 Gilmer Ferry Road
Ball Ground, GA 30107
(800) 858-9888

Cassette Tapes

Budzynski, T. H. 1989. *Relaxation Training Program.* New York: Guilford Press.

More New Harbinger Titles

THE CHRONIC PAIN CONTROL WORKBOOK
A team of specialists in all areas of pain management detail the treatment strategies for managing and recovering from chronic pain.
Item PN2 Paperback $17.95

FIBROMYALGIA & CHRONIC MYOFASCIAL PAIN SYNDROME
This survival manual is the first comprehensive patient guide for managing these conditions. Readers learn how to identify trigger points, cope with chronic pain and sleep problems, and deal with the numbing effects of "fibrofog."
Item FMS Paperback, $19.95

PREPARING FOR SURGERY
Details tested techniques to prepare the mind and body for surgery—techniques that have been found to help decrease the need for postoperative pain medicine, reduce complications, and promote a quicker return to health.
Item PREP Paperback, $17.95

THE DAILY RELAXER
Presents the most effective and popular techniques for learning how to relax— simple, tension-relieving exercises that you can learn in five minutes and practice with positive results right away.
Item DALY Paperback, $12.95

CONQUERING CARPAL TUNNEL SYNDROME
Symptom charts help you select the best exercises for the movement patterns required by your work and restore the range of motion to overworked hands and arms.
Item CARP Paperback $17.95

Call **toll-free 1-800-748-6273** to order. Have your Visa or Mastercard number ready. Or send a check for the titles you want to New Harbinger Publications, 5674 Shattuck Avenue, Oakland, CA 94609. Include $3.80 for the first book and 75¢ for each additional book to cover shipping and handling. (California residents please include appropriate sales tax.) Allow four to six weeks for delivery.

Prices subject to change without notice.

Other New Harbinger Self-Help Titles